FATLOSS
FOR GOOD

THE SECRET WEAPON

TIFFINY HALL

FATLOSS
FOR GOOD
THE SECRET WEAPON
TIFFINY HALL

hardie grant books
MELBOURNE · LONDON

ACKNOWLEDGEMENTS

Strong warrior hugs and many thanks to the awesome Hardie Grant Team, my superstar literary agent Clare Forster, my beautiful family and darling Ed Kavalee.

Published in 2012 by Hardie Grant Books
Hardie Grant Books (Australia)
Ground Floor, Building 1
658 Church Street
Richmond, Victoria 3121
www.hardiegrant.com.au

Hardie Grant Books (UK)
Dudley House, North Suite
34–35 Southampton Street
London WC2E 7HF
www.hardiegrant.co.uk

Copyright © Tiffiny Hall
Cataloguing-in-Publication data is available from the National Library of Australia.
Fatloss For Good
ISBN 978 174270 249 0

Cover & text design by Tanya De Silva-McKay
Cover photography by Peter Collie
Food photography by Marina Oliphant
Styling by Andrea Geisler
Food by Peta Grey & Laura Donato
Props courtesy of After Store, Market Import, Mark Tuckey, Mud Australia,
Safari Living, The Essential Ingredient, The Works, Bed Bath and Table
Colour reproduction by Splitting Image Colour Studio
Printed and bound in China by 1010 Printing International Limited

DEDICATED TO YOU, MY HEALTH NINJA.

CONTENTS

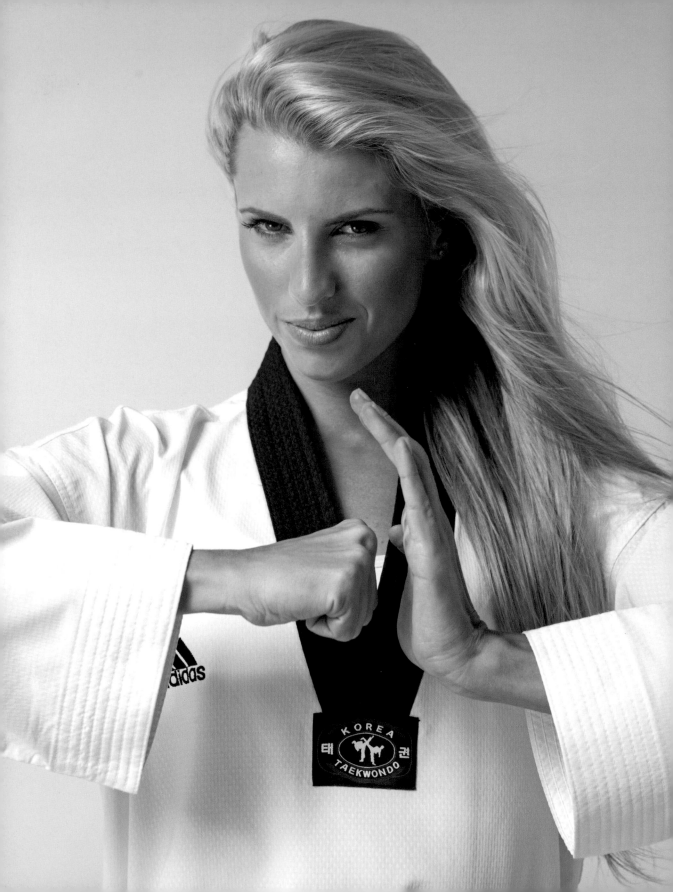

DEAR WARRIORS

I know stuff about brains and how they work and how they change is usually written by doctors and scientists. I'm neither of these things, but you don't have to be a scientist to know that we are controlled by our thoughts. When I joined *The Biggest Loser* as a trainer, I gained a greater understanding of the power of thoughts, and how they affect not only your inner life but also your physical body.

I have been obsessed with the study of the brain (neuroscience) and the changing of the brain (neuroplasty) for years — ever since I realised that when things didn't work out in my life, and I either crashed, became depressed or totally lost the plot, there was always one common thread: my thoughts.

I came to this realisation by noticing my own thought patterns — how they could heal, harm or completely paralyse me, make me triumph or self-destruct. Getting to know my brain and thought patterns, and learning to defend myself against negative thinking and toxic self-talk, has been a long journey for me.

WELCOME, HEALTH NINJAS

I hear ya! I grew up in a family of black belts in a culture of health and fitness. The fridge was filled with luscious, organic goodies, the juicer buzzed every morning at 7 am blending green vegetables, and we all exercised together, in the same outfits, yelling affirmations at the top of our voices. Gees, if I walked past my family stretching in the park and chanting our ninja creed (*'I am a warrior – strong, powerful and centred!'*), I'd hate us too!

Okay, okay. So I grew up ninja. Taekwondo classes every day, being picked up from school by my parents in their taekwondo uniforms (the white pyjamas). I was the only kid at school who had never eaten a fast-food burger. Every lunchtime some kid would ask, 'What's your egg say today?' and before I knew it, kids would be hovering over my lunchbox yelling out the empowering words my mother had written on my hard-boiled eggs.

My father never hesitated to answer the door in his black belt and stare down my first dates. He wore his uniform all over town – to the bank, to the supermarket, even to parent–teacher interviews. He lived his passion for taekwondo every single day, and taught me that being healthy gives you the *kick* of confidence.

My mum can still kick her knee over her shoulder without disturbing her lipstick. She taught me that health was beautiful, so when I hit my teenage years and 'thin was in', as long as I was fit and could sprint, leap, lift, box and throw a mean roundhouse kick – I felt beautiful.

Growing up ninja was fun! Take the ninja out of it and my parents were giving me the greatest education I could receive, teaching me how to defend myself – how to protect my body and preserve my mind. As instructors, Mum and Dad approached taekwondo as self-defence not only against bullies and assailants in dark alleys, but more importantly as defence against junk food, junk thoughts and junk influences.

Everything my parents said could be a bumper sticker: *'Stick to your fitness!'* *'Your health is your wealth!'* *'I've kickstarted my day – have you?'* Life was positive, energetic and active.

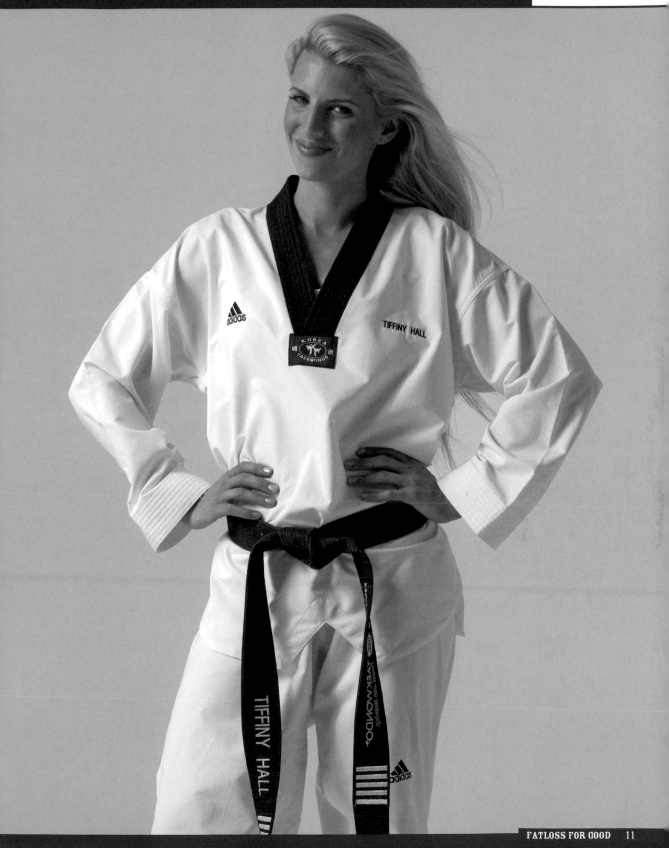

THE POWER OF FOOD!

That was until I moved in with an obese family on *The Biggest Loser*, until then I thought this way of life was normal.

In order to understand the psychology, emotion and power of food, I ate everything they ate, I drank everything they drank and I didn't exercise. In just three days, I gained 4.6 kilos. I ate 1-kilo steaks for breakfast, trays of biscuits, family-sized blocks of chocolate, cheese-wheel sandwiches and buckets of pasta, and washed it all down with beer. Everything I ate during that time was brown and yellow in colour; dead food. I didn't see one bit of greenery on my plate – not even a garnish.

In just one week, my health plummeted. My body was poisoned. I had a chest infection that rendered me on Ventolin and three courses of antibiotics. I felt depressed. The experience taught me that food isn't just about taste, fuel and nutrition – most powerfully, food is all about chemicals. The right food can be medicine. The wrong food can be a drug. Eating dead food that was nutritionally void didn't just hurt my body, it disabled my mind.

I'd grown up thinking that food was about feeding the body, but I was so wrong. Food is all about chemicals that feed your mind. If your mind isn't strong, healthy and happy, then your body has no chance.

After my experience I decided to transform my contestants on *The Biggest Loser* – not by training their bodies, but by training their minds. I would do this the only way I knew how – by turning them into **Health Ninjas**. I knew that my *Biggest Loser* family couldn't change their bodies and become healthier until they changed their thinking. They didn't need new bodies; they needed new brains that could 'think fit, not fat'. They needed to learn the secret to successful fatloss.

Emma Duncan won *The Biggest Loser 2011*, not because I transformed her body, but because I changed her mind. Emma was eliminated in the competition, but she returned having lost more weight than many of the contestants who had never left Camp Biggest Loser. Emma won the competition on the outside, without a full-time trainer or crash diet. She won because she came to understand during her ninja training that permanent change had to happen in the mind first, the body second. She could not have done this without understanding the Warrior Way: that a strong mind leads you to a strong body – a transformed life.

FROM WEIGHTLOSS WARRIOR
TO FATLOSS FOR GOOD

My first book, *Weightloss Warrior*, gave you the tools to change your body – what to eat, how to eat and how to exercise effectively. It showed you how to harmonise your hormones for optimum weight loss, combat cravings and lifestyle assailants, and even trained you in kitchen kung fu. My book helped you to progress from a beginner white belt and train through the different belt ranks to achieve your black belt in health.

Weightloss Warrior received a powerful response to one theme in particular: motivation. First up, I'm sorry to break it to ya, but the Big M doesn't exist. If you want to be a Health Ninja long term, you have to ditch motivation and instead change your mindset, the way you think. I can give you every health tip I know, but if you only train your body, those shiny new tips will never stick.

Losing weight was an important part of Emma Duncan's journey, and the competition of a reality TV show was great motivation, but Emma's path to lasting health wouldn't have been forged with motivation alone. Motivation fades, but creating a healthy mindset lasts a lifetime.

Fatloss For Good will help you change the way you think, so that you're hardwired to be fit and healthy – just like Emma. You'll discover that healthy choices will become automatic through your network of supportive habits – you won't need to rely on discipline or motivation. You will be reborn with a new brain that is happy, healthy and ageless. That's the secret to becoming ninja, from your chemicals to your cortex!

But is the brain capable of change? You bet ya best fly kick on it!

The brain *can* change itself, without medication or surgery, and you can *abso-freaken-lutely* change the way you think. More than that, you can change your whole brain – rewire your mind to think healthy, happy and positively.

If you are a student studying for exams; if you suffer depression or anxiety; if you are addicted to food, drugs, alcohol, cigarettes; if you are unmotivated at work, listless in life, tired all the time, negative about your relationships – then you need this brain boot camp and you need *Fatloss For Good*.

If you are reading this book because you would like to lose weight – 5 kg, 20 kg, baby weight, break-up weight, work weight – then this book is especially for you. I'll show you how you can shed those kilos and rewire your brain so the weight never creeps back on. You will become an automatic Health Ninja!

In fact, this book is for everyone. My training methods on *The Biggest Loser* have been described as 'mental', and you couldn't be more right. Mental training is my speciality. Everyone should train the mind. What I love about martial arts is that it's not so much about fighting physical opponents, but about learning how to fight yourself. Martial arts teaches you to defend yourself against negative thinking and self-destruction.

ANCIENT WARRIORS VERSUS
MODERN PEEPS

Human evolution peaked ten thousand years ago. The ancient warriors of the past lived on instinct – they ate when they were hungry, drank when they were thirsty, fought when they were threatened and slept when they were tired. Always on the move, they protected their families and ate wholefoods, raw foods, nothing processed or refined. And what is the difference between the ancient warriors and us modern peeps? Well, we have forgotten how to listen to our bodies. We have allowed our chaotic lifestyles to strangle our intuition. We have forgotten how to live in accordance with our true nature.

There's a primal instinct within us that is ignited when we are in danger, during competition or when we are faced with stressful situations. Our instinct governs how we act and react.

We are meant to live like warriors, to be on the move for most of the day, to eat only when we are hungry, to use our instincts to govern our food choices, to eat only wholefoods that are fresh and seasonal, and nothing that is packaged. Instinctual eating is so important, but many of us are overweight. The average 21st-century dude isn't strolling along ripped and muscular. We don't have to be fit any more; our families won't be killed while we're out at work, we work hard sitting down and we eat socially, by the clock rather than instinctually.

We've forgotten the warrior race. That's why I'm going to unleash the inner warriors within you. Your inner warriors will help to remind you how to think, feel, eat and move like a warrior.

INTRODUCING YOUR A TEAM OF WARRIORS

Who said you have to fight for your health on your own? I'll show you how you can change your mind and transform your body with the help of a team of Master Warriors.

Inside you lies the dormant power of the Ninja **(STEALTH)**, Samurai **(CONTROL)**, Shaolin Monk **(AWARENESS)**, Gladiator **(STRENGTH)** and Apache **(PROTECTION)**. Who knew!

Fatloss For Good will help you to unleash your warrior power and harness the right warrior at the right time, so you are better trained and skilled to fight your opponent, be it an ambush by a sugar craving, feeling hostage to exercise or the attack of negative thinking.

GO NINJAS – GET YA HEALTH NINJA ON!

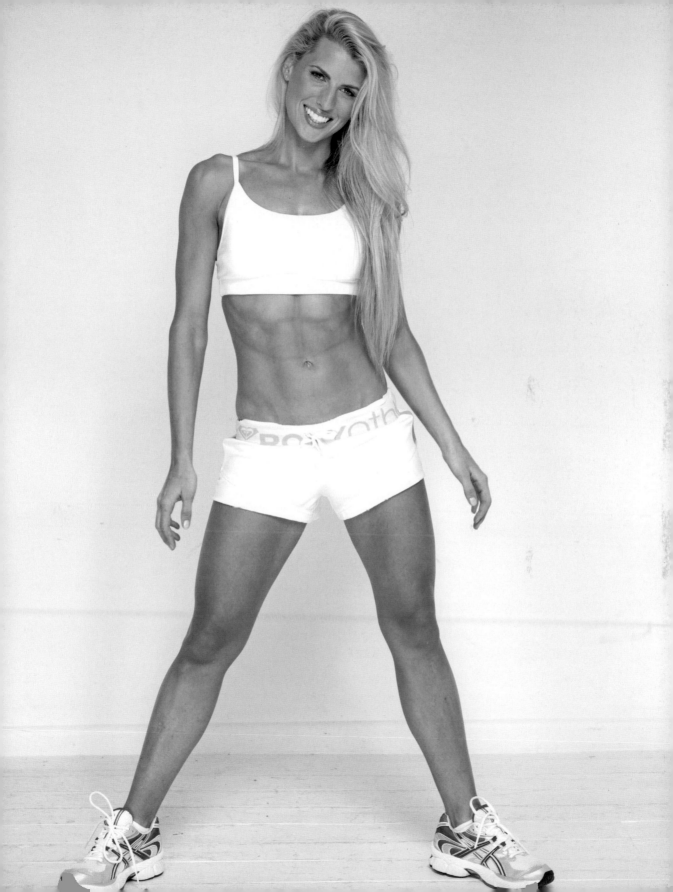

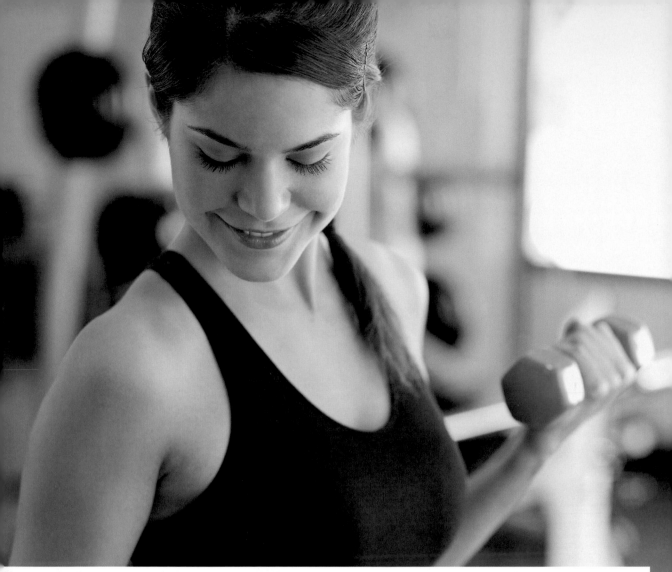

When you have to trick the enemy in order to lose weight, then you gotta be a ninja! Rewire your brain to become a Health Ninja, and you'll shed those kilos.

From inch pebbles
to milestones

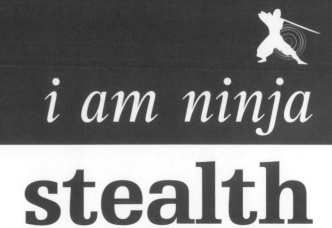

i am ninja

stealth

Ninjas are tricky. The Japanese meaning of nin is stealth, and ninjas are famous for being the best in the business. Armed with bad-ass weapons like ninja stars, ninjas are also masters of psychological warfare, breaking down their enemy's mental defences. Ninjas are known as shadow warriors for good reason, and will fight the fight before you're even aware you've started fighting. I'll show you how to use stealth and deception to short-circuit familiar opponents like cravings and binging by channelling your inner Health Ninja!

Lower the bar

You hear the cliché 'raise the bar' a lot in the fitness industry. Forget it! I'm telling you to lower the bar. In fact, I want you to imagine a bar so low you can step over it. If you want to get your Health Ninja fighting on your side, you have to change the way you look at change. Shrink it so small, you hardly notice it.

Let's say you had never exercised before and I told you to run 21 km a day until you lost 30 kilos. The effort would be inconceivable! But if I told you that your office job was a cardio paradise and that with a tap of a key on your computer you could burn 5 calories (21 kJ), maybe you'd start looking for other ways to be more active in the office too. You would no longer be 0 per cent on the way to your destination, but 20 per cent already there. For habits to happen, progress must be felt – you gotta feel a change is coming!

Confidence karate

On the road to weight loss, life is going to get in the way. Kids will take priority over the gym, you'll get stranded at work once in a while with no healthy snacks and surrender to a bakery walk-by, and there will be training sessions when you're just not that into it. Your weight loss isn't always going to be perfect, because life is never perfect. On these days you have to wave a white flag! There is no way you can improve and keep losing weight when you are slogging away at 16-hour days at the office or your child is sick. What you *can* do is swap your thinking from weight loss to maintenance. On maintenance days, just aim to maintain your hard work: don't overeat, and if you don't have time to exercise, move every little bit you can – at the playground with the kids, make your lunch to-go a healthy wrap and go for a walk on your lunch break.

stealthy ninja

If the thought of losing 7 kg is too daunting, use stealth to minimise your goals, shrink the change required to 3 kg, short-circuit temptation and recognise when a binge is sneaking up on you.

Grow younger day by day

I signed up as a trainer on *The Biggest Loser* thinking it was a weight-loss show. Man, was I wrong! *Biggest Loser* is about saving lives. Eating the wrong stuff robs you of years and makes your brain old before its time. Many of my contestants were more than twenty years older than their chronological age – older than their parents! One of my ninjas, Sarah Jayne, was twenty-nine years old chronologically but her biological age was fifty-three! When my contestants walked out of Camp Biggest Loser, they walked out not only lighter and healthier but also younger. They did this not just by eating healthily and exercising, but by changing their attitude to food – their *fooditude*! – and training their brains.

Change your brain

Keeping your mind active changes your brain – it's that simple. Scientists have proved this by studying rats in a lab. They found that rats in stimulating environments had more neurotransmitters, heavier brains and better blood supply than those in less interesting environments. The same thing happened with lab mice who were given a cardio workout on a treadmill.

Just like those rats, you need to exercise your brain as much as you exercise your body. Flex your mental muscle! Exercising your brain not only makes you smarter, it can also help eradicate depression and feeling low – feelings that all too often lead to eating sugary treats.

Whatever keeps your heart and blood vessels fit also invigorates your brain, including a healthy diet and exercise. We're not talking brutal workouts; if you're nutritionally and mentally balanced, consistent natural movement can be enough. Preserve your brain's health by learning tai chi, Latin ballroom dancing or martial arts. Nothing speeds brain atrophy quicker than being immobilised in the same environment.

Mind Games

The part of the brain that houses our memory of habits and motor skills is called the frontal lobe. We use it to know what we're doing within our environment – in other words, consciousness. The frontal lobe controls our emotional response and our expressive language, assigns meaning to the words we choose and involves word associations. Firming up this part of your brain will help to build new habits, plan your goals and think your way out of health hardships.

keep it real

It's so important to have realistic commitments and goals. Don't tell yourself you are a failure for not losing 5 kg in just one week – you aren't on *The Biggest Loser!* Half a kilo is a healthy, sustainable amount of weight to lose in one week, so aim for that. Commit yourself to 20 minutes of exercise every day and build on that. Or if you are struggling with your metabolism, commit to eating three regular meals a day and then commit two weeks later to eating three proper meals a day. Or even shrink the change by eating a healthy breakfast, then slowly build on eating more mindfully all day.

TIFFINY'S EPIPHANY

Don't try to be the perfect eater or the perfect gym member. Be the best you can be.

'The warrior way is **concentrating on wellness not just fitness.** Pure health is having **compassion for yourself** – sometimes **working on emotional issues** can be just as **important as working out.**'

Welcome to Mind Gym

On our journey as Health Ninjas, building a smart designer brain through Mind Gym exercise is essential to making our health last into our old age.

If you can't remember phone numbers or you take notes compulsively because you don't trust your memory, you need to strengthen your auditory memory. One way of doing this is by rote memorising, which helps strengthen your mind.

Classical education in our grandparents' day relied on a strict regime of rote memorising, handwriting exercises and public speaking. People could debate fluently for hours without resorting to notes, but nowadays many of us would be lost without PowerPoint!

Unless you're a superfreak and can discipline yourself to memorise Latin, work out arithmetic problems and recite Shakespeare every day on your lunch break, you may have few opportunities to systematically exercise your brain on a daily basis. So let's get into the Mind Gym and give our temporal lobes a workout!

NINJAS LOVE BLUEBERRIES

Blueberries are one of the best foods to help memory and learning. They're high in flavonoids, which provide antioxidant protection to promote healthy neurons. Add these blue bubbles of brain power to smoothies, breakfast bowls and salads, freeze 'em an' suck 'em, and bake them in your healthy savoury muffins.

Mind Gym Exercise

1. Learn five cool sentences in a new language: **'Je suis un/une NINJA!'**
2. Discover your 'write mind': when we write something out, our brain converts the words and symbols into movements of the fingers and hands that help us to remember things better. Try learning the lyrics to a song by writing them out.
3. Write down a list of everything you enjoy doing (besides eating!).
4. Dedicate 15 minutes to visualizing yourself achieving your goal. If you want to drop three dress sizes, see yourself in that smaller dress, feeling healthy and exuberant.
5. Practise mind discipline by getting up an hour earlier. Tell yourself the time you want to get up in the morning seven times before you go to sleep. Imagine yourself rising at that time with energy. **And you will**! I promise, ninja!
6. Practise affirmations that don't deprive you of anything: 'I can eat anything I want. But I choose only to eat food that will nourish and strengthen my body and mind.'
7. Write a 'mind mojo' list of all the things you made happen this week because you were in a positive frreeeframe of mind.
8. Take yourself to junk rehab and ditch the junk food for 10 days.
9. Drink a minimum of 2 litres of water every day to keep your brain hydrated and fast thinking.
10. Try to exercise every morning for 40 minutes. Make sure you sweat!

TIFFINY'S EPIPHANY

Anything that flexes your memory, concentration and decision-making faculties can firm up your frontal lobes: conundrums, number quizzes, crosswords, memory cards, problem-solving puzzles.

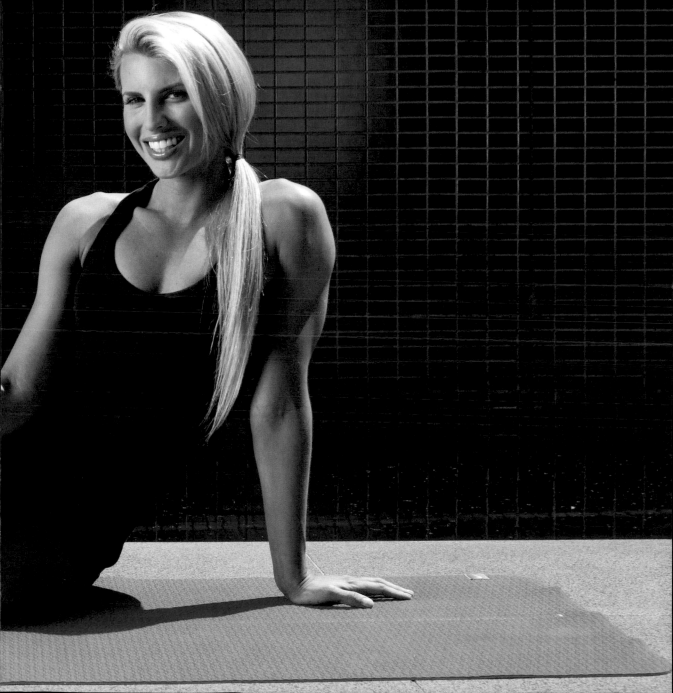

cognitive fitness

Cognitive fitness will help you to build a better, healthier, more supportive brain that looks after you. Just as you can build a bulging bicep, you can build yourself a bigger and better brain by working out in your Mind Gym.

Flex your mental muscle

Flex your mental muscle with puzzles, crosswords and word games. Here's an alpha-numerical quiz to:

(a) use problem-solving by deciphering the mystery code and understanding the provided clue

(b) use decision-making by deciding on which strategy you will use to get back to the original message

(c) give your memory a workout by mentally reciting the alphabet.

Good luck, ninjas!

J R R G M R E: Y R X G R K D Y H D E U D L Q Q L Q M D!

Clue: Each letter in the original message (except the orange Y) has been replaced by another according to this rule: replace each letter with the letter in the alphabet that is three positions before it.

Mental training

It's true: mental toughness can have a colossal influence on success. Mental stamina is what turns a mother of four into a black belt in taekwondo and your old school mate into an entrepreneur. It's not that they have all the athletic prowess or talent – they have the ability to push through; to set a goal and strive relentlessly towards it – they've trained their inner ninja.

In order to become a Health Ninja, you need long-term mental stamina. Ninjas are notorious for their determination – they will do whatever is necessary to fulfil a mission. Here are some ideas to become a Fatloss Warrior with mental training!

- **Overcome fear of failing** – by failing. Make heaps of mistakes and learn from them. If you succeed only 30% of the time, that's awesome! It means you will be failing more often than you succeed, but failing is just a part of life. In fact, you actually learn more by failing than by succeeding. The key is to focus on your mistakes and failures as positive learning opportunities. Ask yourself: 'What didn't go well? How can I do things differently next time to be successful?'

- **Focus on the footsteps, not the finish line:** It's a fact that you have much more control over the process than the outcome. When you want to lose weight, focus on what you can control – your diet and exercise, not the number you want to flash up on the scales.

- **Excuse excuses:** take full responsibility for all of your failures and all of your successes. The world's most successful people never make excuses, and they never take their success for granted.

- **Catapult yourself out of your comfort zone:** When you move outside your comfort zone, you are pushed to grow and develop as a person. So, do some things that are unfamiliar to you: learn something you have never done before, and you will be in a better position to adapt to handling difficult situations with grace.

- **Strengthen your mind with routine:** Routines are one of the most widespread practices among elite athletes, whether in training sessions or during competition. Routines integrate both the mental and the physical, so you steer towards your goal with mind, body and spirit. A routine is a specific way of doing something to stay focused, block distractions and put you in the ideal mindset. It can be a powerful tool, whether it's exercising every morning at 5.30 am before the kids wake up, drinking green tea in the afternoon instead of a latte, carrying an esky of healthy food to work instead of visiting the vending machine, or simply choosing one night a week to switch off the TV and go to the gym instead.

Brain traps

Have you ever made a mistake while playing an instrument, and then kept making that mistake over and over – and the harder you tried to fix it, the harder it was to stop making that mistake? Or have you ever made a mistake while reading out loud and been unable to correct it? When two thoughts merge from neurons firing at the same time, you create a Brain Trap. You fire off a mistake and, feeling more and more anxious to fix the mistake, you only perpetuate the error.

No wonder it can be so difficult to sever bad eating habits! In our minds, we fuse feelings of comfort, relaxation or reward with food. We can't eat without feeling a certain way, and we can't feel a certain way without feeding those emotions with food. This is a tricky situation where you need the stealth of a ninja warrior to help you out with a tactical game plan: small change.

The five-minute makeover

Enduring, successful change is change you can see and feel: that's right, small change. Want to know how to compress change so you don't even notice? With the five-minute makeover, that's how. It's the ultimate stealthy ninja tactic.

So promise your inner ninja you'll spend 5 minutes – a fiver on the treadmill, a fiver cleaning your work desk, a fiver doing laundry basket squats – your inner ninja will start to feel pride in your accomplishment and may even encourage you to spend 10 or 20 minutes on the task. As your confidence builds, you'll keep moving. But the hardest part of getting moving is getting started, so don't start with a marathon – start with five steps in the right direction.

TIFFINY'S EPIPHANY

Any time spent in your Mind Gym strengthening resistance is beneficial, even if only for a minute.

seek HeLP

If you are suffering symptoms of depression, your efforts to lose weight will be sabotaged. It's essential that you immediately seek help as depression is a very treatable illness. According to Melbourne's Royal Women's Hospital, 2 out of 3 women will suffer this condition in their lifetime.

TIFFINY'S EPIPHANY

This is an affirmation I say to
myself when I'm feeling down:
Health is having compassion for
yourself and others.
Love is treating yourself and others
with respect.
Longevity comes from being grateful
for your life and for others.
Passion is living out your
soul purpose.

By limiting the investment you are willing to make, you put less pressure on yourself. Five minutes seems achievable to your inner ninja.

Small wins

Enduring, successful change is change you can see and feel: small wins. In order to succeed, small wins need to have two traits: they must be meaningful and they must be within reach. Remember: your inner ninja is on a mission for instant gratification. Your inner ninja is the reason you can make fast changes but also the reason why you have tried crash diets, magic weight-loss pills and infomercial gym equipment – they tempt your inner ninja with the promise of instant delight!

If you are struggling with an eating disorder, you probably have depression as well. There's no way you will start to make better food choices until you treat your depression. When you start feeling healthier, you will begin to make better choices. You have to feel good to make good choices – it's that simple. That's why I am super against punishing exercise regimes and food-depriving diets. Have a bit of chocolate now and again to feel good and keep you on track. Or sacrifice one hard training session once in a while to watch a DVD.

Feeling good is your top priority, and I've always believed that feeling better comes from eating better.

HOW MUCH WATER SHOULD I DRINK?

Forget glasses. Think jugs! You need to drink around 30 ml of water per kilogram of body weight. That means you should be drinking at least a few bottles of water a day. At my weight, 54 kg, I find 4 litres works for me.

As a start, get yourself a 4-litre water bottle, carry it around with you all day and drink from it for a week. You will be amazed at how *little* water you drink in a day. The 4 kilo weight of the water bottle will give you a good workout, too – if you want to make it easier to carry around, drink up! Measuring your water intake is imperative to understanding your own hydration levels. Unless you get this right, exercise and diet just won't synergise to give you the awesome results.

Short-change change

On *The Biggest Loser*, I had to short change my contestants. Twenty seconds of walking on the treadmill, followed by a 10-second rest interval, soon built to 2 minutes' jogging with 30-second rest intervals, until my contestants could run for 10 minutes without stopping. We celebrated every ninja star throw, every single inch-pebble. And as they moved from one ninja star to the next, they gained confidence and momentum. When they could see and feel change, they were happier to increase the speed or the distance on the treadmill. They began to believe in their capabilities.

TIFFINY'S EPIPHANY

This is an affirmation I say to myself when I don't feel like training: Never sacrifice your mental health for fitness. Never train out of guilt.

eat less = less stress

Remember, our bodies aren't designed to absorb extreme amounts of calories. Our bodies are designed to store energy. Flash back to our hunting-gathering days: our ability to store energy kept us alive on slow days on the hunt or during seasonal crock-ups. The reason you should eat less isn't just because your body is designed to store food. When you eat less, you have less stress at a cellular level in your body, and less cell stress means there are fewer harmful free radicals in your system.

If we had started with a 21 km run, with the aim of dropping 3 kilos a day until they dropped 65 kg in three months, their inner ninja warriors would have given up after a couple of minutes, too exhausted to go on. All I would have heard would have been their favourite excuse: 'Tiff, when I get the urge to exercise, I lie down until it goes away!'

Derail a binge

Negative thoughts and emotions such as feeling hurt, stressed, distressed or depressed create anxiety. If our tolerance to anxiety is low, we can use addictions to quell our discomfort. These addictions can come in the form of gambling, drugs, food and alcohol.

Binge eating is a way of suppressing feelings, burying them so we don't have to feel pain; it's a habit that feeds on negative thinking. The answer is to disengage with these thoughts. Reprogram your thought patterns. Develop reaffirming tracks in your brain, and over time you will learn to disengage from the negative thoughts and feelings, and captain your ninja to stay on your health journey. If your values are to be healthy, in time you'll choose healthy eating over binging because the reaffirming tracks in your brain will lead you to the healthier outcome.

Attack of the giant gelati

When we are dieting, all we can think about is ice-cream. That ice-cream cone is *soooo* big, it's in your face and blocking your vision and your perception of the world. It's all you can think about. 'Ice-cream, ice-cream, ice-cream!' your mind chants. If you mentally heave that ice-cream away, you regain a little distance, but you can still see it blocking your vision and the effort involved in pushing it away only makes you more anxious.

Now here's the thing, and I'm going to be honest with you. Your food addiction will never leave you – no matter how hard you push. The answer isn't to push the addiction away, but to grab hold of it and place it in your lap. If what you are craving is nestled in your lap, then you have a clear view of it in front of you. You regain your perspective and you can see past the craving. You may never be **cured** of your food addiction, but you can learn how to **coexist** with it. You will know it's there, but you can control it.

There are two steps to building up your tolerance to the addiction, so that when it comes screaming at you, you are better able to steer towards your goals and values, rather than towards anxiety: 1. Disengage thought; 2. Self-engage nurture.

TIFFINY'S EPIPHANY

When we have a food addiction, our binge foods become life-size and we can't see past them.

Levels of disengagement with negative thoughts

I'm fat. I might as well binge.
I'm *thinking* that I'm feeling fat and should binge.
I'm *noticing* that I'm *thinking* that I'm fat and feeling that I need to binge.

Disengage thought

When you have a negative thought, disengage from it. When you disengage, that obsessive negative train of thought loses all its steam.

When negative thoughts, pernicious feelings and food addictions strike, think of them as aggressive passengers on a bus. You're the bus driver: if you turn around and yell at them to be quiet, sit down and behave themselves, you will be derailed and crash. When we pay attention to our thought addictions, we strengthen the neural pathways. It will be inevitable that we'll binge eat and give in to our anxiety, rather than move forward towards our goals. Your best bet for avoiding a crash in the pantry with packets of chips is to keep your eyes on the road: don't engage with the passenger in the back, no matter how ballistic or violent they become. You remain the driver, in control of getting yourself to your goals safely.

First off, identify your negative emotion and feeling. Here's one that *every* woman has had – me included. 'I'm fat.' This is a negative thought cultivated from low self-esteem.

The first level of disengagement is to short circuit your thought by labelling it as a thought. Say to yourself: 'I'm *thinking* that I'm fat.' Once you are conscious that your feeling is a thought, the thought loses its aggression in pushing you to act. Just because you are thinking about binge eating, for example, **DOESN'T MEAN YOU HAVE TO BINGE!**

Next, say to yourself: I *notice* that I'm *thinking* that I'm fat. Thinking this way won't help. It's my orbital cortex thingy, not me.' Identifying the thought as a thought, and reminding yourself that you don't have to act on that thought, helps to distance the obsession and bring you back to the present moment. If you are noticing the environment around you, this negative thought will seem futile.

Self-engage nurture

Once you have acknowledged that anxiety is only a symptom of a thought or a feeling, and not a reality, the next crucial step is to refocus on a positive, wholesome, joy-giving activity when you are under attack. Make it non-food though. By *not* acting on food compulsions, you weaken the link between the compulsion and the idea, easing your anxiety. Do something pleasurable in place of the compulsion, and you create a new thought circuit that is gradually reinforced instead of the compulsion – neurons that fire together, wire together.

When you notice a symptom of anxiety, perhaps hunger from feeling hurt, agitated, tired or frustrated, the key is to 'change the channel' of your ruminating thought for 15 to 30 minutes. By concentrating intensely on a new activity, you will be mentally training a new brain pattern away from your obsessive thought. Every time you change your focus, you create new thought circuits.

Trip the mind bandits

Another way to deal with negative thoughts is to make a list of ruminating bad thoughts and label them as Mind Bandits. Don't believe every negative thought you hear! The negative thoughts that automatically enter your head throughout the day make you hate yourself and prevent you from making healthy choices to establish supportive habits and behaviour. They sabotage your plans to eat healthily and to exercise, and can kill self-esteem if you allow them.

Your Mind Bandits were created long ago by certain thought patterns, and when they attack your mind you just can't think of anything else. They then influence your actions and mood.

Your life doesn't make you stressed, depressed or despairing: it's your thoughts that make you feel this way. **You don't have to believe your thoughts.** Once you write them down, then practise recognising them, your Mind Bandits will lose their power. Change your thinking, and you will change your life.

When a negative Mind Bandit blasts in ('I'm a fat mess!'), acknowledge that it is indeed a Mind Bandit. It isn't a true thought. Allow the thought to pass through your mind and instead of binging out of hurt, dismay or will to self-harm, prepare yourself a healthy meal instead, or go for a brisk walk. You are healthy and fit. The numbers on the scale don't mean a thing when you are on the Health Ninja journey. If the negative thought didn't exist, you would feel liberated. And every day that you identify the thought as a Mind Bandit, it loses its power and you are one day closer to being free.

Food feng shui

In today's food culture of supersized *everything*, many of us have lost track of how much food is too much food. Is there no such thing as bad food, only bad portions? Pretty much. Your body is an incredibly resilient machine. You aren't going to get fat off one Krispy Kreme doughnut a month, but you will if you eat six of 'em at a time!

Here are some tried and tested, practical steps to follow on your Ninja Health Journey.

To regulate how much you eat at home, try using smaller plates, bowls and glasses. Then, by filling up half your plate with vegies and fruits, you help yourself reduce the amount of calorie-laden starches, meats and sweets you consume. If you go out to dinner, try sharing two starters with a friend or family member, or take half your meal home in a doggy-bag. Most restaurant portions are far bigger than the average adult needs to eat in a single meal.

Another good tip for in-between meals to take the edge off hunger is to keep snacks on hand, such as a piece of fruit, a serving of black beans or a handful of nuts. This keeps you from eating too much too fast at regular meals.

NOBODY'S perfect

In the past, a lot of my personal failure came from wanting to be perfect. I would make unrealistic demands on myself, based on demands I *thought* people were putting on me. I now realise that much of the time I was training too hard, eating too strictly and striving too dangerously for a standard of perfection that simply doesn't exist. The greatest mental shift I made, and it was only recently, was to realise that perfection doesn't exist.

TIFFINY'S EPIPHANY

Think of your mind as a garden and negative thoughts as weeds. Positive thoughts bloom like flowers but negative thoughts spread quickly, like weeds.

Man-ual feeding

Do you eat the same meal as your man? When you're cooking together, it's easy to have portion distortion – after all, your other half can eat double what you can, more than 1400 calories (5845 kJ) a day, and maintain his weight. He gets away with it because he has more muscle mass, and muscle eats more calories – but us gals? If we match him bite for love bite, we'll blow out. Serve yourself smaller amounts of food. Use a side plate for yourself and a dinner plate for him. Chicks burn 26 per cent fewer calories than dudes. Not fair!

Serial temptationist

One of the contestants on *The Biggest Loser* was terrified of entering her kitchen when she returned home after the show was finished. As a chronic binge eater, she would binge in the same place every night – sitting on the pantry floor. As soon as the sun went down, she would eat until she felt sick. Eating in the dark added over 40 kilos to her petite frame. After leaving the show and losing the binge weight, she was scared that as soon as it got dark, she would binge again. She was petrified of stepping foot in the kitchen and was living off fast food to avoid it. She knew the kitchen was an environmental trigger. She knew that as long as her habit of binge eating was emotionally, neurologically, psychologically attached to the kitchen, she would regain the 40 kg and then some.

How did she face her fear? She smashed through it. She completely demolished her kitchen. She blew up the pantry and redesigned her kitchen with tiny cupboards to store canned essentials, not a huge pantry that could house processed foods and was big enough for her to sit on the floor and eat in the guilty dark. She bought a new fridge and stocked the kitchen with 'naked foods' rather than packaged foods stacked with artificial ingredients. Fresh food was what she needed, along with a fresh slate to commit to a new habit. She took a risk, and now she has kept the weight off. She has no more fear of entering the kitchen and enjoys cooking up the healthy *Weightloss Warrior* recipes.

HOW BIG IS A PIECE OF MEAT?

The portion size for most meats is the size of a deck of cards, or the size of a chequebook if we're talking about fish. When looking at meat, I always use my fist as a guide. I know my stomach is as big as my fist, so it makes sense to eat a piece of meat that's no bigger than my fist or the palm of my hand. So if you have visions of a steak covering three-quarters of your plate, you should probably share that T-bone with a mate.

Beware platefuls of spaghetti and meatballs, or casseroles (I know, yummo!). Many people fill up their plate with foods like this and call it a meal. In reality, it should only take up at most a quarter of your plate – after all, it's meat! Meat meat meat! Just because it's a bit fancy doesn't mean you can eat more if it.

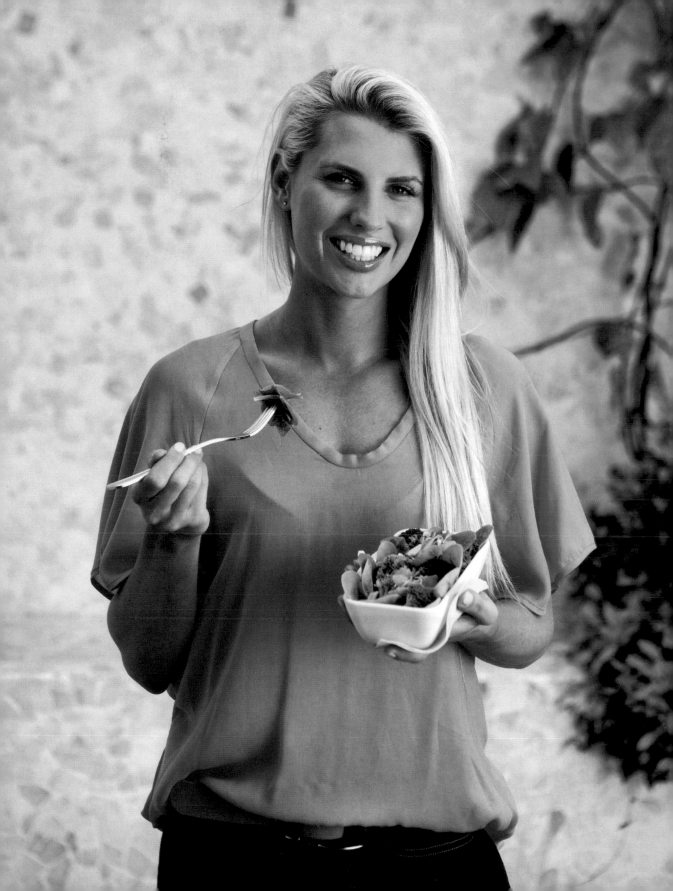

Ninja stealth against portion distortion

- Ditch the candles – when the lighting is dim, you're more likely to linger over your food.

- Blue walls are proven to suppress appetite, and blue lighting makes food look less appealing – warmer colours, especially yellow, have the opposite effect.

- Use smaller serving bowls, and never eat out of pasta bowls – the bigger the bowl, the more you'll stuff it full.

- Tall tumbler glasses look harder to drink out of and may put you off. Stick with short, deep glasses so you can really chug the water down and drink athletically.

- If you know you often overeat, train your eyes to size up the correct portion size by eating off smaller plates. Hulk-size plates and bowls encourage bigger portions, so keep them saucer size. To begin with, eat off a side plate – your stomach will adjust to the new portion and so will your eyes. Instead of eliminating dessert, swap a bowl of ice-cream for a cup of ice-cream. Small plate = smaller portion. Look for plates no more than 25 cm in diameter and limit yourself to teaspoons and dessert forks. Even use teaspoons to load your plate, and they definitely make the best dessert spoons. Smaller utensils = smaller bites.

Trick triggers

It's *so* important to identify your triggers and to disarm them with the stealth and subterfuge of a ninja. Ninjas are kings of trickery. Their clan was formed from the poor who had to survive by any means possible, often resorting to thieving and trickery. If you want to trick a trigger, then walk in the stealthy steps of a ninja.

Environmental triggers

Often, we're so wrapped up in our problems that we can't see how simple the solution can be. For example, think about your daily routine. Does your commute to work include driving by the local doughnut shop or walking past those greasy food carts? At work, do you routinely walk by the vending machines on your way to the toilets? The solution - take a different route to work or make the trek to the bathroom on the other side of the office. By finding ways of managing your particular situation, you can control which temptations you come into contact with and, over time, become stronger at resisting.

THE ART OF CELLULITE DEFENCE

- Avoid zero-fat diets

- Don't cut down fat too low – make it 10 per cent or more of your total calorie intake

- 1 tbsp of flax or Udo's Choice oil blend can fix you up with essential fatty acids for the day.

- Use a nonstick spray instead of coating your pans with oil. And when you spray, don't put a fire out – 2 seconds is all you need.

- Butter is empty calories – no essential fatty acids, no good fats – consider eliminating it all together. Instead of spreading butter on rye toast, use avocado or natural peanut paste spread.

- Eliminate margarine

- Cut down on processed meats such as bacon, salami and sausages

- Buy lean cuts of meat

- Eat salmon and trout – fabulous fat!

- Trim visible fat from meat

- Remove skin from poultry

- Eliminate commercial pâtés, dips and pastry-based products

- Use low-fat dairy products

- Muffins aren't healthy snacks – muffins are cakes and full of evil fat

- Minimise your intake of snack foods such as manufactured cakes and biscuits, chocolates, potato chips and takeaway food

- **Only eat what you cook – this is eating naked**, stripping your food of all processing and packaging

- Embrace avocados, nuts, seeds, olives or natural peanut butter in moderation

- Salad dressings with olive oil or balsamic vinegar are best – avoid all other squirts

- Banish fried foods – they won't unleash any inner warriors. Over time you'll stop craving them, and soon your powerful new warrior physique will stop you from ever wanting them again!

TIFFINY'S EPIPHANY

Regular exercise not only protects the cells in your body, it also makes them better at kicking butt.

TRIGGER TRICKS

- If the couch triggers overeating, watch the news on the treadmill at the gym.

- Start saying no to commitments that trigger you to feel overwhelmed and make you turn to food for comfort. The 'no' muscle is one of the most important muscles to keep in tip-top condition!

- Record your measurements once a month and avoid the scales – they only trigger guilt or frustration.

- If driving triggers you to eat out of your glove box or perform criminal Drive Buys for fast food, keep your hands on the wheel and your mind involved in listening to an audio book.

- If you are always running late and skipping breakfast triggers you to rely on the vending machine at work, prepare breakfast the night before: fast-lock bags of muesli, milk, berries – mix at work. Boil eggs. Make savoury muffins from pumpkin puree to have with morning tea.

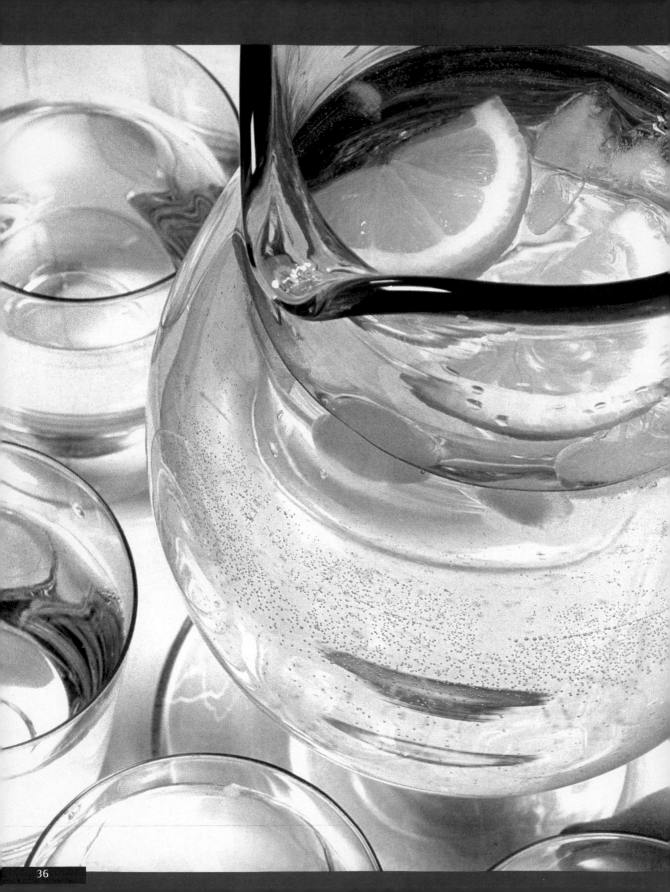

TRIGGERS

- Skipping breakfast and eating muffins for *lunchfast* at 1 pm
- Vending machines
- Wheeling your trolley down the confectionery aisle at the supermarket to get to the milk down the back
- The tea and coffee *and biscuit* station at work

- Eating free samples at bakeries
- Going to a party on an empty stomach and destroying the finger food
- Skipping the gym for a date
- Snacking in front of the TV
- Eating in the car
- Devouring Maltesers at the movies

The best way to disarm triggers is to EOL — eat out loud. Keep a food journal, and write down *what* you eat and drink, *when* you eat and drink, and *where*. Log the exercise you do, and the calories you chew. Doing this will inhibit calorie amnesia and also illuminate your triggers. Perhaps you don't eat enough? Or you eat too much after exercising? Maybe you eat sweet foods only in meetings?

Are you drinking food?

The brain is the only part of us that is constantly active. It processes all the information it receives from different parts of the body, as well as the info it receives from daily exposure to the external environment. In other words, the brain uses heaps of energy! It receives energy from two sources: food metabolism — the formation of sugar — and water supply — the conversion of hydroelectric energy.

When you're feeling stressed, your body becomes dehydrated because your brain is working overtime to deal with your stress. The reason we tend to gain weight is simple: we eat to supply the brain with the energy it needs to work on our stress! However, when we eat, only 20 per cent of that food energy reaches the brain. If you don't get up and do something, the remaining 80 per cent will gradually become stored in your body as fat. Your brain doesn't need food energy at 3 pm when you're chained at your desk counting down to 5 pm; your brain needs *water energy*. Your body will store food energy in case of starvation, but it won't store water in case of dehydration.

PLATING UP NINJA STYLE

- A serve of meat = your fist
- ½ cup pasta = a tennis ball
- 1 cup cereal = your fist
- 30 g cheese = 4 dice
- 1 piece of fruit = your fist
- 1 tbsp butter = half a ping-pong ball
- 1 tsp butter = the tip of your finger
- 1 pancake = a CD

TIFFINY'S EPIPHANY

We aren't camels — we're elephants!

The **samurai code** is all about respecting your **healthy** inner self. If you have self-respect, you'll have the **self-confidence** to eat well, exercise **mindfully** and treat yourself nice so you can lose weight and keep that weight off.

Not only will you become a Health Ninja, you'll become a **Samurai Warrior!**

2

Change your **destiny**

i am samurai

control

IN CONTROL

One of the few things we can control in our life is how well we treat ourselves through healthy choices and empowering thoughts. This is the philosophy of the samurai. Once you gain control of how you feel, how you eat, how you think and how you move, you will feel more in control when you step into the outside world.

While the ninja fights in the shadows to win by whatever means possible, the samurai fight in the open. Honour is paramount to samurai warriors, and they never resort to subterfuge. The samurai live by their code of honour, and are loyal, devoted and respectful.

Your inner samurai will encourage you to honour yourself and your weight-loss goals with healthy habits. They'll help you to sever old habits that don't support your healthy new way of life, and nurture a sense of respect and loyalty towards the healthy you that lies inside. Being a samurai will help you to close your eyes to those freshly baked brownies your colleague brings in to work, and ignore that pile of chocolate bars on the counter when you line up to pay for petrol at the service station. Go on, get ya Samurai Warrior on!

The samurai versus ninja brain

Ninjas and samurais have been enemies since the dawn of time. Sneak attacks, poison, seduction, spying – these methods of war are all fair game for the ninja, but being rational and ethical, the samurai loathe those tactics.

Your brain is half ninja (emotion) and half samurai (rational) in the way it approaches your health – no wonder it can be tricky to referee! While the ninja clan hungers for instant gratification, the samurai will fight on with right on their side.

Picture the emotional side of your brain as a clan of black ninjas and your rational side as a single silver samurai warrior wielding an enormous sword. Whenever there is a surprise ninja attack, the samurai is almost always outnumbered and overpowered. If you've ever slept in, overeaten, texted your ex, skipped the gym, tried to quit smoking and failed, abandoned a gym class or lied to your personal trainer – your rational samurai has been attacked by ninjas. We've all been there! When change fails, you can often blame those naughty ninjas.

Your inner samurai provides the focus for your actions, while your ninjas fuel your passion and energy. Without the samurai you would lack direction, but without the ninjas you would lack the hunger and drive. To achieve long-term change, you have to appeal to both teams of health warriors.

The three-hour day

Treat every three hours as a new day. Forgive yourself for a slip-up and start again in three hours' time. One slip-up doesn't mean you have to write off the entire day. Doing this will prevent binging and self-destruction, and also put a cap on the guilts. When you are healthy and fit, you are rewarded with a body that can deal with the effects of succumbing to temptation once in a while. A treat or a little naughty food once in a while will never make you fat, but binging will. Treating is okay, feasting is not.

How to pacify your ninja clan

You will never transform a ninja into a samurai, but what you can do is change your environment and so reduce conflict. Some habits have nothing to do with you at all, but are the result of your surroundings. If you are trying to lose weight, it's vital to make sure your environment is supporting that goal; your kitchen, home, car, workplace, supermarket and your support network.

The best way to achieve immediate results is to change your biochemistry. How do you do this? With food! Eat the right stuff and you'll feel immediately brighter, lighter and more energetic; it takes longer to see the benefits of exercise. Your ninja clan want immediate self-gratification, remember, so eating yourself lighter is your best shot.

Self-control is exhausting

Want to know the secret to lasting health and weight maintenance? Lean in …

All those health gurus who tell you to eat this and not that are telling you to exercise self-control over every meal you eat, every workout you do, every single thought and desire. Managing this kind of self-control won't work forever. Controlling your ninjas is exhausting!

You are totally wearing out your inner samurai by fighting ninjas all day, exhausting the mental muscles needed to bring about change. Exercising willpower and self-supervision is so fatiguing, it's no wonder you binge after going on a diet, or eat ice-cream with a ladle after a 30-day cleansing regime.

The road to health may not be as effortless and automatic as tying your shoe laces, but there are techniques to living a healthy, vivacious life: after a bit of practice, your reactions to enemies (negative thoughts) and assailants (alcohol, cigarettes, sugar, junk food) will be automatic. Together we can build up our reflexes. *Ay yah!*

perfect isn't perfect

Health doesn't have to be perfect: if you aim to be a Stoic Samurai 80 per cent of the time, and give 20 per cent to your Naughty Ninja, then you will continue to be healthy and lose weight. But if you make a mistake and give into a mini binge, don't wait for tomorrow to start being healthy again.

TIFFINY'S EPIPHANY

Shrink your day to a window of three hours and make every Three Hour Day count.

TIFFINY'S EPIPHANY

You can't fight your emotions – accept them. You can't banish your desires – so accept them.

You won't bring peace to mortal enemies like the ninja and samurai overnight – after all, these guys have been at each other's throats for yonks – but what you *can* do is retrain them to fight for your health harmoniously. The ninja brain will *always* be fuelled by emotion; the samurai brain will *always* exercise control and rationale – this doesn't mean they can't fight the same fight with different techniques. You can use stealth to outsmart emotional triggers and traps, and samurai swords to cut through new choices and forge more supportive habits.

CHOCOLATE VERSUS RADISHES

A study conducted on hungry college students invited them to participate in what they thought was a 'food perception' test involving highly distinctive tastes and food memory. Feeling hungry after not eating for at least three hours, they were asked to enter a room that smelt delicious – the researchers had just baked a fresh batch of chocolate-chip cookies. The students were presented with two bowls: one was filled with a sampling of chocolates, along with the fresh-baked chocolate-chip cookies they could smell; the other bowl held a bunch of radishes.

Half the students were instructed to eat two or three cookies plus some chocolates, while the others were instructed to eat the radishes. The poor radish-eaters nibbled on their rabbit food while watching enviously as the other students devoured the plump, still-warm cookies.

At that point the 'food perception' test was officially over and a new group of researchers took the students through a second, supposedly unrelated study into who was better at solving problems. The students were presented with a series of puzzles that required them to trace a complicated geometric shape without retracing any lines and without lifting their pencils from the paper. In reality, the problems were designed to be unsolvable. The researchers wanted to see how long the students would persist in pursuing a difficult, frustrating task before they gave up.

The 'untempted' students, those who had eaten the chocolate-chip cookies, spent nineteen minutes on the task and made thirty-four well-intentioned attempts to complete the exercise. The radish-eaters gave up after only eight minutes, and they managed only nineteen attempts to solve the puzzle.

Why did the radish eaters quit? They exhausted their supply of self-control, that's why.

samurai
newsflash
Super small. Rather than starting with a zero-carb diet and a two-hour run, choose a glass of water instead of a soft drink or swap white bread for wholegrain. Eating naked and taking small, consistent steps will make big changes happen effortlessly.

Control self-control

The best way to deal with the conflict between reason and emotion is to recognise when the emotional ninja onslaught for junk food is about to begin. Rather than send out your rational samurai to fight for your health, why not say, 'Thank you ninjas for reminding me of the toxic food that I once ate and made me feel disgusting.' In acknowledging the thought, you disarm the ninjas' greatest weapon: subterfuge. The samurai wins!

SHADOW-FIGHTING SAMURAI

My father was an Olympic coach when I was growing up. When I was aged 16, he was preparing his fighters for the Sydney 2000 Games. I would go to our dojang to watch the elite players train, and I was always surprised to see them fighting without an opponent, shadow sparring aginst themselves. My father was a big believer in the power of the mind to improve performance: visualisation.

Every student who joined our taekwondo clubs had to master shadow sparring. My father believed that how you envision yourself fighting in your mind will exactly mirror how you will fight on the day of competition.

In the lead-up to the Games, I remember my father challenging one of his female fighters to fight for three minutes without breaking her concentration – to do all the fighting on the taekwondo courts of her mind. He wanted her to move around the court fighting, kicking, screaming, scoring as she would do on fight day at the Olympics. When I first watched her do it, she could only make it to 30 seconds. Six months later, she made it to three minutes.

I thought my dad was crazy but at the 2000 Olympics, Lauren Burns won a gold medal – the first medal for our sport in history. I knew that my father's visualisation techniques had something to do with it.

We don't tend to pay much attention to our parents when we're teenagers, but after I witnessed Lauren's spectacular win, I realised the importance of knowing how to spar with ourselves. In our mind's arena, we shadow fight each other every day.

Self-control is exhaustible

That's right – psychologists have discovered that self-control is an exhaustible resource. It's just like doing push-ups at the gym – the first one is easy when your muscles are fresh, but with each additional repetition, your muscles grow fatigued until you can't lift yourself off the ground. The radish-eaters had depleted their self-control by resisting the cookies, so when their ninjas started fighting the puzzle test, their response was *it's too hard, no fun, we suck!* Their inner samurai could only fight the ninja clan for eight minutes, while the cookie-eaters had a fresh, untaxed samurai to fight the ninja. This is why fad dieting never ever works. A fad diet will always make your ninjas more powerful against a samurai.

SAMURAI STAT: PICTURE THIS

Scientists have studied the effect of learning a new motor skill on the brain area involved with movement. Two subjects were instructed to play a five-finger piece on a keyboard connected to a computer, practising for two hours a day over a period of five days. The subjects' brain areas corresponding to finger movements were measured, both before and after the study. Sure enough, those motor areas grew significantly – as we know, nerve cells grow with use. But what was remarkable about this experiment was that the second subject practised only in his mind. He didn't lift a finger to actually play the keyboard.

The subject who *imagined* himself playing the piano had the same change in his brain as the subject who physically played the piano each day! His neural circuits were stimulated and grew solely in response to his imagination.

My father's belief in mental rehearsal got me thinking: if I could imagine myself enhancing my sport with my father's Jedi mind trick, what else could I think *better*? In my final year at school, I aimed for a near-perfect score of 98.75 to get into Melbourne University. Applying the same mental rehearsal to my studies as I did to my taekwondo, I visualised the achievement of this score: I imagined the questions on the exams in detail, and imagined myself writing down my answers to those questions with confidence and clarity. And you know what? I achieved the exact score I needed: 98.75, not a point higher, not a point lower. This remains one of my greatest achievements. Not because of the high mark, but because it was the first time in my life I was able to *visualise success*.

When we try to change things in our lives, we need to tinker with habits and behaviour that have become automatic. Changing them requires careful supervision by the samurai. The bigger the change you're looking to make, the more it will drain your self-control.

What I'm proposing is that we ditch the whole self-control/willpower angle and opt for something more basic. Not change, but **choice**. I'll give you the best choices to make, show you how to distract your ninja clan from dangerous situations, and little by little, we'll retrain our ninjas to walk in harmony with the samurai. Good health will become automatic, and not an issue of self-discipline. Deal?

TIFFINY'S EPIPHANY

Change is hard not because people are lazy, but it's because they wear themselves out. What looks like laziness is often exhaustion. Self-control burns out.

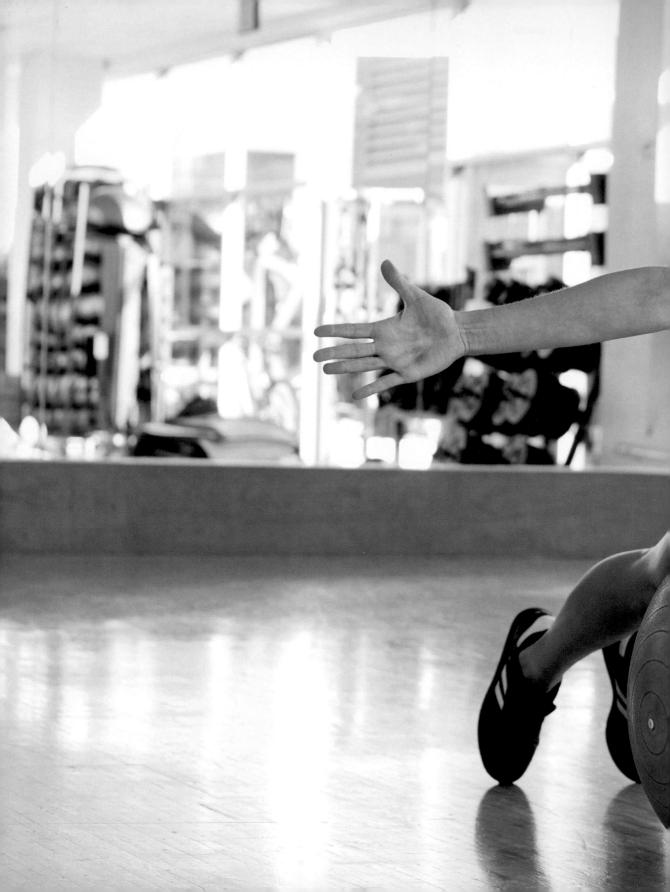

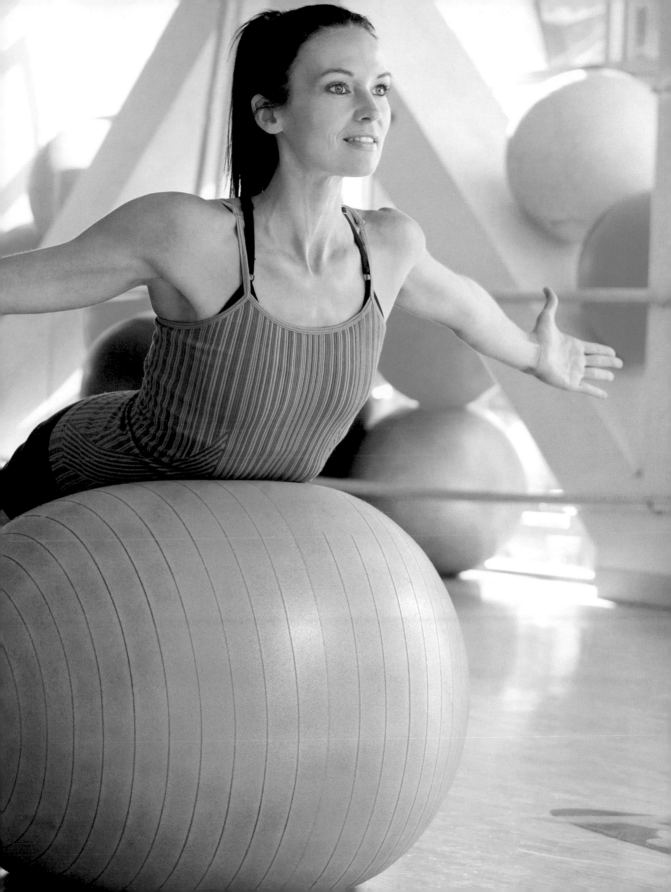

Change your habits

Want to know the question I am asked most often? It's this: what's the secret to staying motivated to lose weight? Ha! Motivation doesn't exist, remember! Consistency is the answer.

Consistency is critical if you want to make a habit — maybe exercising regularly or eating naked — become automatic. To become a habit, it has to be done every day.

If you want to learn a new language, you gotta speak it every day. Becoming healthy and fit is just like learning a new lingo — you have to immerse yourself in it and commit. Directing your focus to the task for any amount of time will help to cement your new habits.

THE MAGIC #30

Three to four weeks is all it takes to make a habit run on auto.
The following Samurai Warrior plan can help make that habit stick over the next 30 days.

Start a journal: Start a journal on the first day of the month to log your progress and bright flashes of success.

Don't try to be perfect: Sorry ninjas, success won't be immediate. Try your best, but expect a few bumps along the way. Life ain't perfect, and neither are you. Accept this and we'll all live happier ever after.

Detailed repetition: The more consistent your habit, the easier it will be to stick to it. If you want to start exercising, try doing it at the same time, at the same place for your 30 days. Replicating the time, place and circumstances can make new habits stick more easily.

Reminder: Forget iPhone reminders — human reminders are the best! Ask a friend or your partner to gently remind you just how far you've come if you start to stray. Around two weeks into your commitment it can be easy to forget.

Do it for yourself: Don't worry about being selfish and putting yourself first before your family. Unless you are happy and healthy, they won't be happy either.

Change negative thoughts: Try this great technique for changing bad thought patterns: when you start to think negative thoughts, use the word 'but' to interrupt it. 'I'm no good at this, but if I work at it I might get better later.' I 'but' myself all day, and it works!

Visualise successful patterns of behaviour: Visualise yourself performing a bad old habit. Next, visualise yourself pushing aside that bad habit and pursuing the alternative. Finally, end that sequence with an image of yourself in a highly positive state. See yourself picking up the cigarette, see yourself putting it down and snapping your fingers, then visualise yourself running and breathing freely. Do it a few times until you automatically go through the pattern before executing the old habit. If you feel like binging, see yourself eating an entire bag of lollies; imagine how it will make you feel and the consequences. Then imagine throwing the lollies away.

Don't take yourself too seriously: This isn't life or death. Treat your new habits as an experiment. Withhold judgement until after a month has past, and use it as an experiment in behaviour. Experiments can't fail – they just have different results, revealing what works and what doesn't for your inner samurai.

Warrior scrolls: A piece of paper with a resolution on it isn't that important, but writing down that resolution is. Writing forms clarity. Clarity will help keep you on track to achieving your goal.

Know the benefits: Familiarise yourself with the benefits of making a positive change. Read some books that detail the benefits of regular exercise. Have your biological age tested so you know how old your body is in comparison to your chronological age. Have a fitness test or a full medical. Get the stats so you know your starting point. Exposing yourself to realistic information about the downsides of not making a change will give you added motivation.

Coach: Find someone who will support your journey and motivate you when you feel like quitting. Motivation can come from phone calls, powwows, exercise buddies, your family, partner, a good friend or a professional. Whatever your goal – remember you don't have to go it alone.

Banish temptation: Design your environment so it won't tempt you over those first 30 days. Remove junk food from your house, cancel your cable subscription, throw away the cigarettes and cancel any social functions that you know will tarnish your new habit. Once the habit is formed you will be strong enough to deal with temptation but in the initial stages you must self-protect.

Replace lost needs: If you are giving up something to pursue your new habit, make sure you replace any nurturing you've lost. If watching television was relaxing, you could take up meditation or reading as a way to replace that same need. Relaxation doesn't have to be sedentary. You can have active rest through walking, swimming, cycling or yoga.

Evolve with role models: Spend more time with people who model the habits you wish to mirror. A recent study found that having obese friends made you more likely to become fat. The people you surround yourself with are a reflection of who you will become. If your family is unhealthy, kickstart a health journey together. To change your habits, you have to change your eating, drinking and movement culture.

Monday to Tuesday: Make your habit day-to-day.

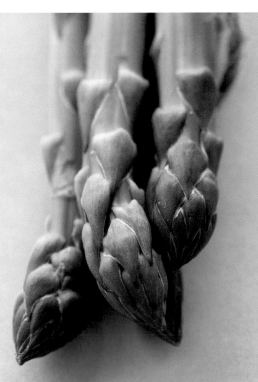

'Don't be afraid of change. Change is only making a different choice. A change of feeling is a change of destiny.'

The chemicals in our brain can make us feel a certain way. That's why it's important for Health Ninjas to get their heads around mental chemicals!

Endorphins – pleasure and pain
Endorphins are the chemicals you want to have on your side when you make food choices and choose a type of exercise – treat 'em bad, and they'll repay you with loss of control. The Runner's High is no myth: exercise boosts your endorphins.

GABA – calming and relaxing
GABA is an amino acid that helps regulate brain excitability. Low levels of GABA have been found in people with psychiatric disorders such as depression and anxiety. Green tea boosts GABA and aids focus.

Serotonin – happiness, bliss, peace of mind
Serotonin regulates everything from sleep and appetite to impulse control and sexual desire. It soothes us when we feel stressed or threatened, and plummets when we binge on sweet things. Signs of serotonin depletion are insomnia, cravings, muscle aches, impulsive behaviour, moodiness, irritability and low self-esteem. Stabilise your insulin levels with vitamin B, nude foods and exercise.

Dopamine – motivation, drive, mental focus.
You might be dopamine deficient if you feel fatigued, apathetic, have difficulty losing weight, feel unmotivated and depressed. Vitamin B, omega-3 fatty acids and herbal therapies such as ginkgo biloba and St John's wort can boost your dopamine levels.

Energy factories

The economics of energy are like good investments: spend it wisely and you will get even more of it.

Energy is a renewable resource within our bodies, as well as in the world around us. We aren't aware of it, but there are millions of tiny factories inside of us that are constantly producing the energy that we need to keep us going. Known as mitochondria, these energy factories are found inside every cell in our body, in varying numbers, depending on how much energy that particular cell needs to ninja up.

And which part of the body do you think has the highest concentration of mitochondria? That's right, it's the brain, which uses a full 20 per cent of the body's main fuel – glucose blood sugar. The rest of the body can use other sources of energy, like protein or fat, but the brain relies solely upon glucose as power. If that energy supply starts running low, our blood sugar drops and our

TIFFINY'S EPIPHANY
Give yourself a ninja star of self-esteem: when results are consistent, fast and measurable, you don't need discipline. Yippee!

body's alarm bells start ringing in the quest to find food! When we eat high sugar diets, our brains experience these drops in sugar levels and send us searching for food more often – this is experienced as cravings or anxiety.

DO THE MATH

Most brain functions are dependent on energy from sugar – that's why we've developed an appetite for sugar when we feel brain drained or tired. Our bodies convert stored carbs for energy, followed by proteins, and finally fat. Fat takes longer to metabolise: each gram of fat transfers 9 calories (38 kJ) of energy, while each gram of protein or sugar provides only 4 calories (17 kJ) of energy. That's why when good fat is metabolised, you feel less hungry.

Eat naked

Your brain is just as affected by toxins and chemicals as your body. That's why samurais choose to *eat naked*.

Eating naked is the simplest way I've discovered to eat healthy. You might be thinking, 'I'm not stripping off to eat!' Don't worry, that's not what I mean! Eating naked is about stripping down your food so it isn't clothed in packaging, and therefore isn't processed. I *know* that naked eating works for health, *dramatic* weight loss and to reverse your biological age. It makes sense to eat *real food* – the kind of stuff that rots if it isn't eaten, that our ancestors would recognise, that isn't chemically enhanced or preserved.

Most of the food on offer today is no longer naked – it's fake and processed. Processing depletes food of nearly all its fibre, vitamins and other micronutrients, leaving you with pure carbohydrate, which our bodies have to digest and turn into sugar, a drug that affects our brain chemistry.

The speedy rise in blood sugar triggers an equally fast release of serotonin, flooding us with those floaty feelings that pacify us after a sugar spree. This boost is not only short-lived, it may also lead to further depletion of serotonin levels. You see? When we binge, the crash makes the 'I'm feeling awesome!' chemicals drop way down, and that's why we experience guilt after a binge, or even depression. Consistent binge eating can contribute to mood disorders.

SHADOW-FIGHTING SAMURAI

Best brain foods

- Almond milk, unsweetened
- Almonds, raw
- Asparagus
- Avocados
- Beans, black, pinto
- Beets
- Blackberries
- Blueberries
- Broccoli
- Brussels sprouts
- Capsicum
- Carrots
- Chicken, skinless
- Cranberries
- Egg whites
- Grapefruit
- Greek yoghurt
- Green tea
- Kiwi fruit
- Lemons
- Lentils
- Oats
- Olive oil
- Peas
- Pomegranates
- Red grapes
- Salmon
- Soybeans
- Spinach
- Strawberries
- Sweet potato
- Tofu
- Tomatoes
- Tuna
- Turkey, skinless
- Walnuts

Mind your health, mind your family

Did you know that the food you eat today, the lifestyle choices you make right now, will determine the genetic outcome of your future children?

Genes carry information from one generation to the next, instructing the body how to build itself, beginning with the first cell division and continuing for the rest of our lives. You can't alter your genotype, but how your genes are expressed, how they show up in your life (like switch cancer on or off), is actually quite variable.

The expression of your genes is influenced by a host of different factors, such as how much your parents exercised, their chemical exposure to alcohol, preservatives and tobacco, and mental or emotional factors such as the effects of long-term stress or cultivating positive emotions. Everything you absorb into your system has the potential to change your gene expression. In other words, the future of your family can be served on a platter.

Try these top Health Ninja moves to improve your health and your family's future.

TIFFINY'S EPIPHANY

It's all about self-nurture, not self-torture. Treat yourself as your BFF.

EAT IN ORDER

Eat the low-calorie portion of your meal first – salad, vegies and soup – and eat slowly. Eat the meats and starches last – by the time you get to them, you should be full enough to eat smaller portions.

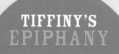

TIFFINY'S EPIPHANY

Eat healthily, do some exercise and change your *fooditude!*

JUST SAY NO!

If you think a sneaky bickie here and there won't hurt, remind yourself that two cream biscuits at morning tea and two in an office meeting in the afternoon can deliver up to 420 calories (1754 kJ). A kilo of body fat equals 7000 calories (29,225 kJ), so if you snack this way for two months, you will gain a kilo without even noticing.

WATCH YOUR FRUCTOSE INTAKE

Fructose leads to increased tummy fat, insulin resistance and metabolic syndrome. Even the humble apple has the same amount of fructose as two teaspoons of sugar. Limiting sugar is the best way to regulate your metabolism, since fructose sabotages our appetite control and instantly turns to fat!

BREAD WINNER

If you want quick weight-loss results, give bread a break. Supplement bread slices with cos lettuce and wrap your fillings in a salad leaf or two. For breakfast, serve your eggs on a thick slice of eggplant.

WHEN IT COMES TO CHOCOLATE, BE A SMARTIE!

Drink cocoa made with skim milk to satisfy chocolate cravings. Swap to dark chocolate from milk chocolate. Add chocolate protein powder to some natural yoghurt or a hot bowl of oats.

'A bad habit is first a spider,

then a thread,

then a rope,

and finally a chain.'

BE A PLATE PERFECTIONIST

Remember to use smaller serving bowls, cos the bigger the bowl, the more you'll stuff it.

SET OUT YOUR OWN FOOD LAW

Like stocking your cupboard with nuts rather than bickies. Most importantly, become aware of your cravings, and when you do eat, eat mindfully.

EAT FROM YOUR FRIDGE, NOT FROM YOUR PANTRY

If you are eating mostly from the pantry, then you aren't eating naked. Pantry food is processed; fridge food is fresh.

SWEAT IS THE NEW BLACK

Even if you only have five minutes to bust a move, do it! You may only burn 150 calories (626 kJ), but you'll burn a further 200 calories (835 kJ) from the metabolic boost and after-burn. You'll kill a whole muffin out of those five minutes of movement. Score! The rule for intensity: if you're not sweating, you're not working hard enough.

SPEAR YOUR BREKKIE

Asparagus spears are a great way to start the day because, being a diuretic vegetable, they reduce fluid retention. The stems are stacked from stalk to tip with nutrients and minerals, and they taste great with rye toast, tomatoes and poached eggs.

EAT OFTEN

Every three to four hours to keep blood sugar levels stable.

ALWAYS EAT BREAKFAST

After fasting overnight, your brain needs fresh fuel. If you don't break the fast and eat breakfast, you starve your body and you starve your brain.

EAT A DIFFERENT TYPE OF PROTEIN AT EACH MEAL

Including eggs, dairy (yoghurt, cheese), beans and other legumes, vegetables, fish, chicken and red meat.

LIMIT FRUIT JUICES

You are better off eating the whole fruit – you need the fibre to balance the rich concentration of fruit sugar (fructose) that stores as immediate fat.

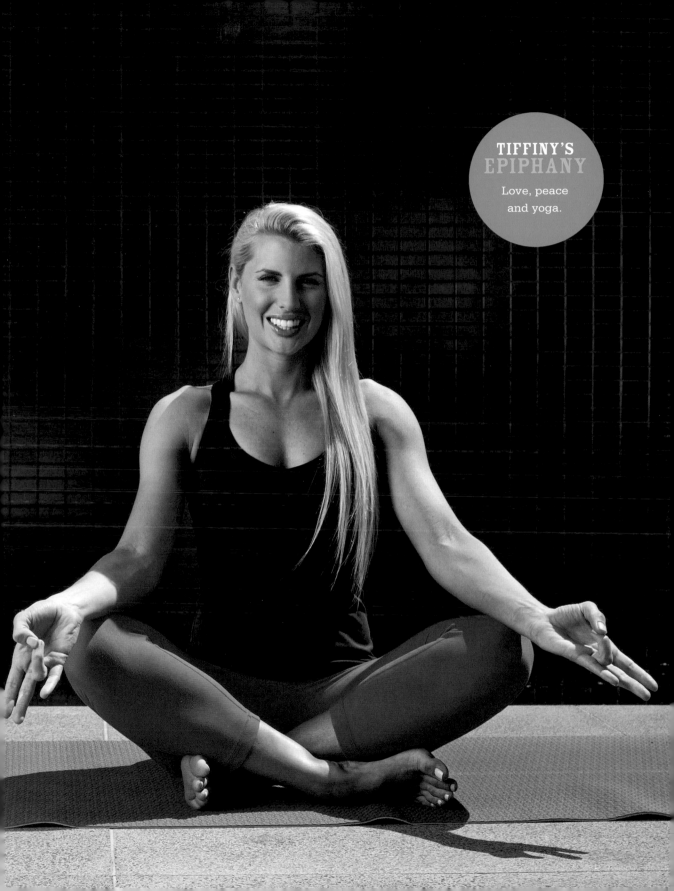

TIFFINY'S
EPIPHANY

Love, peace
and yoga.

ROLL OUT OF BED & INTO KITCHEN KUNG FU

Sure, you've heard the advice to 'eat brekkie first thing'. But consider: if you sleep for six to eight hours and then skip breakfast, your body is essentially running on fumes by the time you get to work. And that sends you desperately seeking sugar, which is usually pretty easy to find ...

KNOW YOUR WHITES

1 cup (250 ml) of milk =

Full-cream milk: 163 calories (681 kJ), 9 g fat

Reduced-fat milk: 125 calories (522 kJ), 3.5 g fat

Non-fat skim milk: 105 calories (438 kJ), 0.3 g fat

Soy milk: 165 calories (689 kJ), 7.5 g fat

Vitasoy Lite: 65 calories (221 kJ) s, 2 g fat

Oat milk: 165 calories (689 kJ), 7 g fat

Almond milk: 105 calories (438 kJ), 1 g fat

Food rainbow

One of the best ways to be healthy is to eat across the colours of the rainbow.

Red

A tomato a day keeps the skin doctor away! Tomatoes are the best form of self-defence against environmental damage to your largest organ − your skin − thanks to the key ingredient, lycopene, an antioxidant. Lycopene levels are highest in cooked tomatoes − so ditch the cream carbonara for bolognaise or napoli, for more protection and fewer calories too.

Orange

Sweet potatoes, carrots and pumpkin contain beta-carotene, which your body converts into wrinkle-vanishing retinol to seal your skin from evil sun damage and make you look goddess gorgeous!

Yellow

Healthy fats aid the body's absorption of lycopene and other nutrients, so try a cap of fish oils, flaxseed oils or an omega-3 supplement − good fat makes you more fabulous!

Green

Green spinach leaves can make you younger? Sure can! Spinach not only builds biceps, it's soaked in vitamin A (beta-carotene) to enhance skin cell regeneration. These super leaves fight inflammation and free-radical damage (villainous wrinkle attackers), thanks to their high concentration of antioxidants, in particular lutein, which helps makes your eyes dazzle. What a samurai! Spinach will do all this for you with only 7 calories (29 kJ) to a cup. And it's not only spinach that carries all these beauty-boosting powers − collard greens, kale and Swiss chard will beautiful your inner samurai too!

A TALE OF TWO FRIDGES

A friend of mine couldn't lose weight because her housemate kept stocking the fridge with tempting junk food she could never resist. I suggested she should buy her own fridge and only eat from that. So she did. Despite the odd look of two fridges sitting side-by-side in the kitchen, my friend took great pleasure in going to farmers markets to stock her fridge with luscious organic produce and she shed the weight easily. She stuck to the warrior rule of only eating from the fridge, never from the pantry (processed foods), and never opened her housemate's fridge, which she termed the 'fat fridge'. How far are you willing to take your commitment to health to disarm your environmental triggers?

Blue

Blueberries are stacked with antioxidants called anthocyanins. They help defend you against the attack of premature ageing and dehydration by defusing the free radicals that make your skin look tired. Throw the cosmetic enhancement of vitamin C into the mix, and the little blue gems stimulate skin-plumping collagen too, working overtime to turn back the clock. These guys pack a real beauty punch, with no assault on your waistline at less than 100 calories (418 kJ) per cup!

Violet

Purple grapes are rich in Vitamin C. They aid blood circulation, so your body is perennially Health Ninja ready — hydrated, rejuvenated and invigorated.

Brown

Chocolate often cops the blame for blemishes, but it's the *type* of chocolate you eat. Chocolate contains flavonoids, potent antioxidants for sun protection, and it enhances blood flow to help keep your skin young and supple — who knew: this relationship saviour and mood enhancer is also a beautician! Forget the cheap stuff that's packed with sugar. Opt instead for chocolate containing 70 per cent cacao (= more antioxidants) to honour your inner samurai. Also, if you're a self-confessed chocoholic like me, steer clear of buying entire bars and buy individually wrapped chocolate drops instead. Snack on one or two chocolate drops a day, or swap them for a low-sugar hot chocolate to crunch the craving. Even better, buy raw cocoa nibs (there's no bitterness, I promise) — these guys are great to snack on. Roast them, and your kitchen will smell like a yummy chocolate factory.

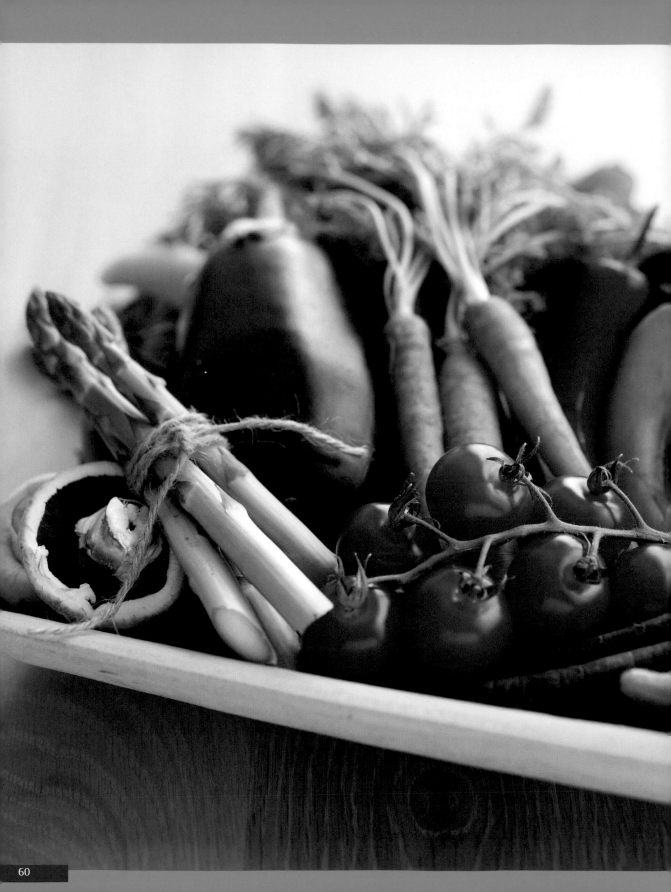

Fibre: the samurai sword

We all know our bodies need calcium for bones, vitamin C to fend off colds, and chocolate to save relationships. But we can't forget using the samurai sword of fibre to cut out the risk of cancer, heart attack and high blood pressure. Most importantly, fibre keeps you full, and is a friend to those of us travelling the Warrior Way. But this doesn't mean you have to eat food that tastes like cardboard. Try these Samurai Steps to sneak fibre into your foods:

- Shower ground flaxseed over your favourite cold cereal, or stir a few spoonfuls into a cup of yoghurt or oats – 2 tablespoons equals close to an extra 2 grams of fibre.
- Choose fibre spreads such as mixed nut paste or almond butter to lather on wholemeal toast – 2 tablespoons adds 2 grams of fibre, along with a healthy dose of heart-protecting fats and vitamins like E.
- Try to eat brown as much as possible. If you don't like wholewheat bread, choose rye bread – a slice has almost 2 grams of fibre, twice the amount found in white bread.
- Tower your burger stack with a sesame-seed bun instead of white bread – sesame seeds add half a gram of fibre per burger.
- Choose burritos instead of tacos – flour tortillas have more fibre than taco shells.
- When it comes to beans and Mexican, say, 'Please may I have some more!' Half a cup of beans adds grams of fibre to your meal.

DITCH aBC & CHECK medications

- Go steady on Alcohol, Bread and starchy Carbs.
- When choosing protein, eat protein that swims before it flies: fish before chicken.
- Certain medications can cause weight gain, including the Pill. Check with your doctor or pharmacist to see if there is an alternative medication without this side-effect.

Low-fat slices

Slice your fat with the best low-calorie bread buys:

Calories per average 40 g slice of bread

Traditional white = 105 calories (438 kJ)

Gluten-free low GI = 75 calories (313 kJ)

Sourdough bread = 88 calories (367 kJ)

Spelt bread = 80 calories (334 kJ)

Wholemeal/wholegrain = 65 calories (271 kJ)

Raisin toast = 97 calories (405 kJ)

Rye = 65 calories (271 kJ)

Soy, linseed = 100 calories (418 kJ)

Pumpernickel bread = 55 calories (230 kJ)

Calories per individual rolls etc

Baguette = 600 calories (2505 kJ)

Roti = 160 calories (668 kJ)

Dinner roll = 105 calories (438 kJ)

Hot cross bun = 230 calories (960 kJ)

Knot roll = 140 calories (585 kJ)

Wholegrain roll = 249 calories (1040 kJ)

1 cup of croutons = 150 calories (626 kJ)

Croissant = 280 calories (1169 kJ)

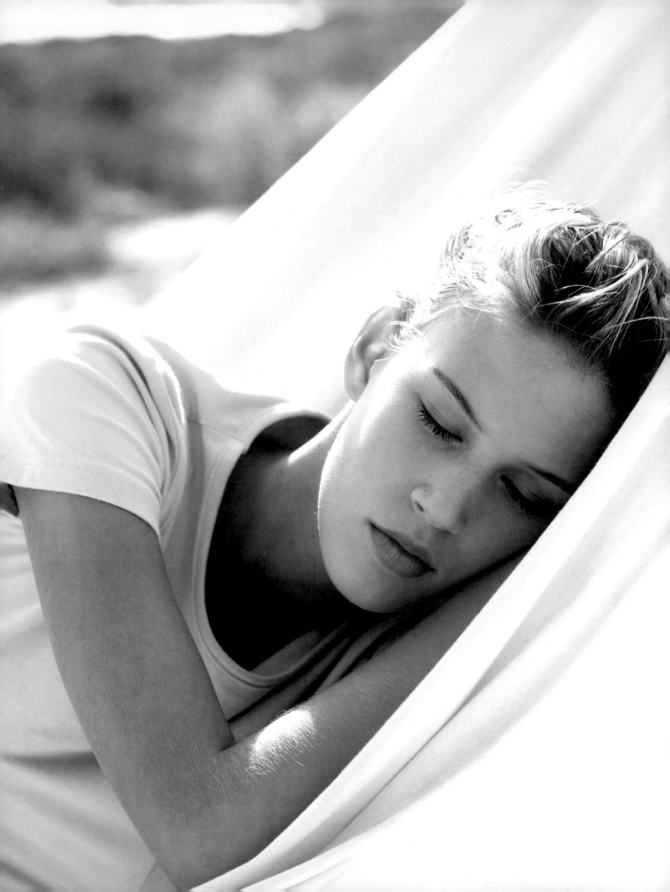

- Toss half a cup of chickpeas into a pot of your favourite soup to suck up the flavour and spice up an added 6 grams of fibre.
- Stir spinach into your favourite pasta sauce – it will pad out your fibre by more than 2 grams.
- Prepare wholewheat or spinach pasta instead of the white stuff for a 5 gram bonus.
- Cook broccoli, cauliflower and carrots, and you'll ingest 3 to 5 grams of fibre per serving – as much as twice what you'll get if you eat them raw, since the heat makes fibre more accessible.

samurai move

WEAPONS OF MASS REDUCTION

- Metric measuring jug
- Metric measuring cups and spoons
- A ruler
- Small plastic containers for measuring single portions of pasta sauce or curries
- Electronic food scales – the only place scales are good for are in your kitchen

SLEEPY SAMURAI

Most adult samurais need seven to eight hours' sleep per night. Bad sleep patterns can trigger anxiety and depression, and increase stress. Too much stress, and fat doesn't burn; not enough sleep, and muscles don't repair. You can't force yourself to fall asleep but you can control when you get up in the morning. If you wake up at a consistent time each day, you will find it's easier to fall asleep more easily and naturally at night.

- Choose a wake-up time that you can live with, say between 6 am and 8 am. Regulate your sleep patterns by getting up within an hour of that time every day (even on weekends!).

- See if you can stretch out your nights by gradually allowing yourself an earlier bedtime. Go to bed fifteen minutes earlier each night until you wake at your desired time without an alarm.

- Keep yourself to that schedule for at least two or three weeks. When you consistently wake refreshed without an alarm you've discovered the amount of sleep that's perfect for you. You may notice you need more sleep in winter and less in summer.

- Use a calming herb such as valerian, passionflower or chamomile in tea before bed.

- Stop stimulating activities at least thirty to sixty minutes before bed. Replace it with something soothing and calming such as reading.

- Watch antihistamines and cold remedies. Look for pseudoephedrine on the label or the letter D after the brand name – they can keep you up.

- Gradually reduce your intake of caffeine until you no longer have trouble falling asleep.

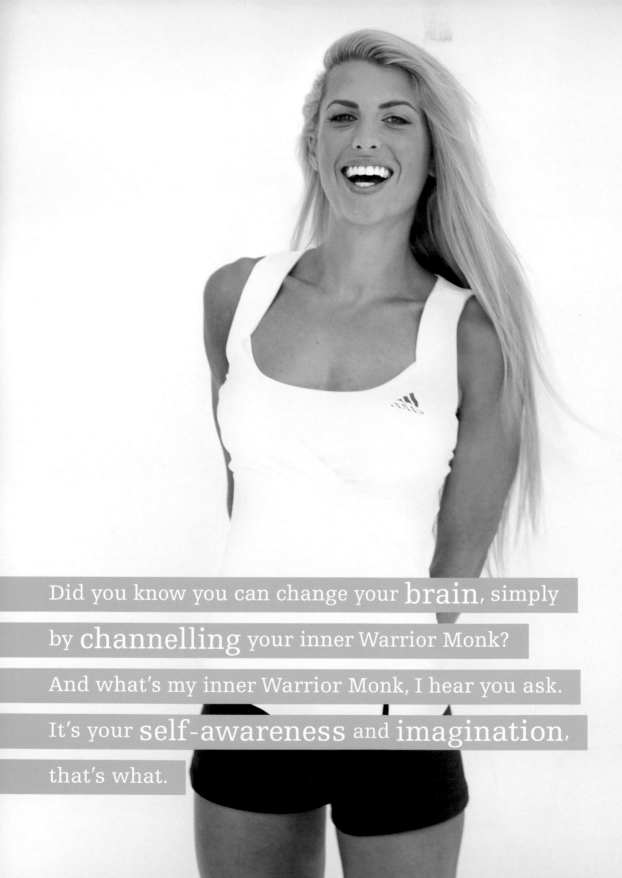

Did you know you can change your **brain**, simply by **channelling** your inner Warrior Monk? And what's my inner Warrior Monk, I hear you ask. It's your **self-awareness** and **imagination**, that's what.

3

Rewire your **brain**

i am shaolin monk

awareness

Here's an example of repetition that works: as soon as you wake up each day, touch your toes – or as close as you can get to them as possible. Touching your toes each day, just once or twice, will increase your flexibility by 27% in just six weeks.

MONK MOMENT: NEW PATHWAYS

Your brain grows new neural pathways in as little as a week. Repetition makes them concrete, so those fresh neural pathways will still be in place after a couple of months, even if you have a break.

I'm not monking around! If you want to lose weight and develop a healthier relationship with food, it's time to practise thinking, eating and moving *healthy*. With repetition and your inner Warrior Monk on your side, you'll make these new habits stick. You won't need motivation; you'll have wired your brain to automatically think healthy.

The mind has the power to heal or harm, to put 10 kilos on or rip 15 kilos off. Your mind can build you a glittering mansion or a dusty old shed. It can help you lose weight and help turn back the clock, making you feel younger by improving your health.

Mental health plan

What forces us to reach for junk food, to stay in bed instead of getting up to exercise, to think negative thoughts and limit our potential? It's not about our bodies – it's all about the power of our minds. The quality of our life is the quality of our mental health. It's that simple.

Okay, you can go on a diet for a few weeks and improve your skin. You can sign up to the gym and change your body through exercise. But the motivation to continue will be fleeting. What *will* keep you exercising, eating healthily and striving for success isn't a matter of motivation, but mindset.

Train the mind

Train the mind, then the mind will train the body. That's my philosophy, and that's how I helped Emma win *The Biggest Loser*. Rather than setting out to change my contestants' behaviour or bodies, I rewired their brains. They walked out of Camp Biggest Loser over 15 years younger than when they arrived, because they had become healthier in both mind and body

MONK MOMENT – EMMA DUNCAN

'I lost 62 kg with Tiffiny – my weight-loss percentage was almost half my starting weight! The most important part of earning my black belt in health was mastering how to train the mind, and then allowing the mind to train my body. I used Tiffiny's Mind Gym just as much as the dojang. This has helped me to keep the weight off and now I can have Little Ninjas!' – **Emma Duncan, age 25, Winner of** *The Biggest Loser* **2011**

In order to learn the technique of positive thinking, we need to learn how to interrupt our negative thought patterns. I reckon Positive Thinking should be taught at school, along with Maths and English. After all, there's no point knowing anything if we limit our potential to use that knowledge.

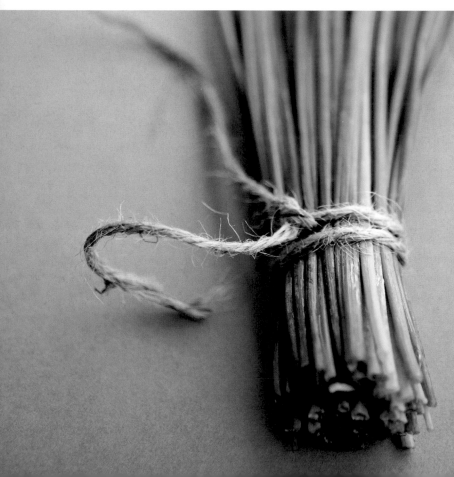

Don't eat junk food,

don't think junk thoughts.

Get ya zen on

Imagining an act and doing it aren't all that different. When you close your eyes and visualise a butterfly, your brain is activated just as if you were actually looking at that butterfly. Brain scans show that the same parts of the brain are activated by the action and the imagination.

Studies have proven that you can imagine your body stronger. A study group who undertook a finger muscle exercise was compared to a group who only imagined doing the exercise – and you know what? At the end of the study, the physical group had increased their muscular strength by 30 per cent, as you'd expect, but the others had increased theirs by 22 per cent.

The explanation lies in the brain's motor neurons that program movements. The neurons responsible for stringing together sequences of instructions for creating physical movements were activated and strengthened by the mental exercise, resulting in increased strength when the muscles were actually used.

No wonder mental practice is often used in sport! Shadow boxing is really like playing mental chess. In fact we all practise mental rehearsing – when we memorise answers for a test, learn lines for a play, or prepare for a race – but because we don't do it systematically, we fail to monopolise its power. We need to monopolise our inner monk!

Harnessing the power of mental practice is the first step on the Healthy Ninja path to weight loss. Use visualisation to be your best, mentally and physically, in your mind, and the reality will follow.

Power Monk

A healthy mind is a beautiful mind, and it all begins with your inner Monk Warrior.

We create our reality through our thought patterns. That's why negative thoughts are so powerful. Unexamined repetitious thought patterns can become real, all too painfully so. But it doesn't have to be this way. Not if you call upon the strength of your inner warriors to become aware of those thought patterns and understand that they are causing you harm.

When we are aware of our thoughts, we can see them for what they are – thoughts, not real. We can question their validity, reflect upon them, and choose whether or not to believe or act upon them. **You don't have to believe every negative thought you hear!**

TIFFINY'S EPIPHANY

Your weight isn't only a symptom of the junk food you eat and how little you exercise – more importantly, it's also a reflection of how you think.

SHAOLIN MONK MOVE

Soviet human rights activist Anatoly Sharansky used mental chess to survive 400 days spent in freezing, dark solitary confinement. Political prisoners often fell apart mentally because they didn't stimulate their brains, but Sharansky played mental chess over the months until he was released. He went on to become a cabinet minister in Israel, and later beat world chess champion Garry Kasparov. He truly harnessed his inner Shaolin monk!

Pull the plug on negative thoughts

We allow negative thoughts to become repetitious by giving them our attention. This is dangerous. When you give thoughts 'airtime' in your mind, you bring them into existence and they can affect your choices and actions.

It's like hearing a hit song played over and over on the radio: the more you hear it, the more the tune gets stuck in your head. And so, the more you listen to a negative thought like 'I'm fat', running round and round in your mind, the more you reinforce that thought through repetition, the more it is strengthened and the more the neural pathway becomes ingrained. Very soon, you will make the thought appear to be true by believing in it.

Many of our negative thoughts are based on two things: fear of the future and a belief that we are somehow flawed. The answer lies in good health: if you are healthy, your self-esteem will improve and you'll see fewer flaws in your physical body. When we are healthy, we live more in the present and less in the future or the past. This is called mindfulness.

Mindfulness helps you to stand your ground in the face of an emotional or mental storm. It builds a foundation of inner strength that can keep you from being helplessly rained on by a bad mood or by negative thoughts about how much you weigh. The mental awareness of mindfulness will disrupt the pattern of a mental storm and deplete its energy.

The best way to interrupt a negative thought pattern is to change your behaviour. Bring yourself back to the now by doing something different from your usual reaction to a negative mind storm. As soon as a negative thought thunders, change your body language. Stand up if you're sitting down, turn on the car radio if you're driving, go for a jog or a walk, or just run up and down the stairs or hallway if you're at home.

When you change how your body moves, you will change the way you feel, and this feeling will change your current thought patterns and focus. Short-circuiting negative thinking in this way will shock the usual negative emotional reactions you experience entirely offcourse.

Mindful eating with your inner monk

If you've put on weight, it's because you've extracted your mind from your mouth! Unconscious eating leads to overeating, and overeating leads to fat gain. Eating mindfully will help you to become healthier and lose fat forever.

Here are some ways you can eat mindfully:

- Set aside specific meal times to dedicate to eating healthy, wholesome and flavoursome food.
- Prepare food in advance. Write out a meal plan for the day. Enjoy shopping for groceries and preparing your meal, knowing it will make you think, act and feel energised.

shaolin monk move

What you say to yourself in your mind is who you become. Your thoughts are your destiny: they forge your brain of the future.

- Before you take your first bite, notice the feeling in your belly, the sense of anticipation, the changes in your mouth as it prepares to receive the food.
- Keep your awareness on your stomach, noticing especially when you are beginning to feel satisfied and have eaten enough. See if you can stop eating before you have the sensation of feeling full.

Stimulate your senses

We all know that thoughts can be positive and negative. Inside your brain there is a war of nerves going on. Picture your A-Team of warriors all defending you.

Every thought in your mind is fighting for space – but become aware of your inner warriors and you'll begin to notice them fighting against self-defeating enemies like negativity and binging. The best way to help your inner warriors win against a negative thought attack is to self-nurture by bringing yourself back to the present moment.

How do you do this? Through your awareness of the senses, that's how. Repeatedly bring yourself back to earth by initiating one of your senses, and in each instance describe your experience: if it was a colour, what colour would it be? If it was a person, who would it be?

sнаоlin мonк move

MIND CONTROL
When negative thoughts hit, say to yourself: 'They are just thoughts, not reality. I can control my thoughts and therefore control my reality.'

MONK MOVE: BE A SENSATE SENSEI

To beat food addiction with the help of your inner Shaolin monk, exercise your five senses:

Visual: Lock eyes on something around you and describe how it makes you feel. Bring yourself back to the visual world.
Tactile: Hold an ice cube or a handful of frozen berries and concentrate on the texture, the temperature. Bring yourself back to the physical world.
Sound: Listen to your favourite song and pick out an instrument. Try to listen only to that single instrument. Bring yourself back to the auditory world.
Smell: Light a candle. Close your eyes and breathe in the scent. Bring yourself back to the world of scent.
Taste: Keep frozen grapes or blueberries in the freezer. Suck on them to bring yourself back to the world of taste.

TIFFINY'S EPIPHANY

Whatever we give our attention to gets stronger, for what we think, we become. Pay attention to what you pay attention to!

If you only see the unhealthy part of yourself, then that part of you will become enlarged and distorted. To regain control over your thoughts, try to place more focus on what *isn't* wrong with yourself.

It takes a mere 17 seconds to shift your focus to a positive thought such as being healthier. Try it: as your focus on good health becomes stronger, your intention becomes clearer. With practice, you will be able to hold your focus on that goal for a period of 68 seconds, after which time your mind will be strong enough to make a healthy choice.

When you repeatedly return to a positive thought, and if you're able to maintain that thought for at least 68 seconds, then it will become a *dominant* thought. Once you have a dominant thought, it will become habitual.

Three important words

There are just some words that Fatloss Warriors hate to hear:

Change – yuk! It makes me feel as if all the flavour, sweetness and colour are about to be sucked out of my life.

Habit – yawn! It conjures up all the boring self-help books my Dad encouraged me to read through my teen years to make me 'effectively efficient'. No thanks!

Discipline – run! Say the word to a health-seeker and they think you're going to spank them with a Zero-carb bible every time they reach for something sinful like a mint macaroon!

Right. So here we are, wanting to lose fat for good, and deep down in our guts, sitting next to that guilty choc-chip muffin, is the sneaking feeling that our long-term success depends on three words we hate: CHANGE. HABIT. DISCIPLINE.

It's natural for us to resist change. Smokers keep smoking, coach potatoes keep watching tv, we keep getting fatter. So how do we change things when we don't want to change? The answer: change your environment and change your mind.

Step one: change your environment

We achieve fantastic results on *The Biggest Loser* because we take the contestant out of their comfortable environment and place them in a controlled situation, one that's compatible with achieving weight loss. Change the situation and you can change the individual.

I'm not suggesting you abandon your family home or quit work to change your environment. But you *can* learn how to outthink your emotions and change situations that don't support your Health Ninja journey to weight loss. How? By recognising the all-important triggers.

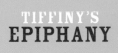

TIFFINY'S
EPIPHANY

Eat with your mind,
not with your
tongue.

Be trigger happy

There are approximately 558 words relating to emotion in the English language, and a whopping 62 per cent of them are negative. Just as Eskimos have 100 different words for snow, it turns out that negative emotions are our snow, that bad is somehow stronger than good.

The key to success as a Warrior Monk is to be mentally and physically prepared for any situation. Think of yourself as being on a mission: if you take the time to think ahead, you can come up with ways to combat every situation.

Triggers don't have to be negative. Creating your own healthy triggers can be a positive ritual that you use as part of your health routine. They are integral to forming successful habits – athletes perform tuck jumps before a race, some people chew gum instead of smoking a cigarette, others can't go for a jog unless they have their iPod with them. Find your own triggers that work for you.

Trick your emotional triggers

First off, let's identify your emotional triggers:

- Anger
- Happiness
- Restless
- Sadness
- Loneliness
- Discouragement
- Fatigue

- Stress
- Boredom
- Excitement
- Frustration
- Anxiety
- People – are there certain people in your life who make you want to eat?

Now that you've identified 'em, try this as an alternative way of dealing with your emotional hunger, other than with food.

Make a list of the things that make you feel good. When you feel those negative feelings rising to the surface, take out your cue card and do something that makes you feel positive and empowered. Your list could include:

- reading
- going to the movies
- meeting up for a coffee
- listening to music

- taking a walk
- having a lovely long bath
- going shopping

Even something as simple as calling a friend on the phone can help calm your ravenous feelings and provide nourishment in a more positive and nurturing way.

shaolin monk move

Eating 'fun foods', or treats, in moderation will never make you fat. But binging will. Resolve your emotional hunger and you will stop the binging. Stop the binging and you will banish fat forever.

Habitat triggers

Not only do we need to detox our minds of negative thoughts, and our bodies of chemicals and preservatives, we also need to cleanse our lives of environmental triggers.

- Go through your kitchen and throw out all the junk food and processed garbage. You don't have to fight if the enemy isn't sleeping in the house!
- Don't buy these foods any more, just eliminate them from your shopping list and kitchen entirely.
- Reacquaint yourself with your local farmers market and supermarket: find the healthy sections, and try to avoid the aisles containing the foods that make you feel powerless. And never shop on a hungry stomach!
- If there's a vending machine in the kitchen at work or if the cafeteria features frightfully fattening foods, stay away from these places. Go for a walk for lunch and eat your meal on the move.
- Pack yourself a Working Warrior lunch in an esky.
- Bring healthy snacks from home to stash in your desk.
- Check out other danger zones: your glove box, office drawers, your wardrobe, the kids' 'reward' shelf, eating from the pantry, eating standing up in the kitchen, social events, work lunches, sitting in front of the TV and being bombarded by ads for junk food.

TIFFINY'S EPIPHANY

I exercise before breakfast because it sets me up for the day mentally and spiritually. I feel more powerful all through the day if I move my body as soon as I wake up. Exercise is my trigger for feeling in control, in body and mind, all day.

Step two: change your mind to transform your body

You can send a drug addict to rehab, but what happens when they leave? For you to change your life and lose weight, you can't just change your environment – you have to change the way you think.

Remember that ninja and samurai fighting it out in Chapter Two? Our brain has two minds: we have a rational mind that wants to eat healthily, and we have an emotional mind that craves chocolate every time something upsets us, like when that spunk didn't text us back.

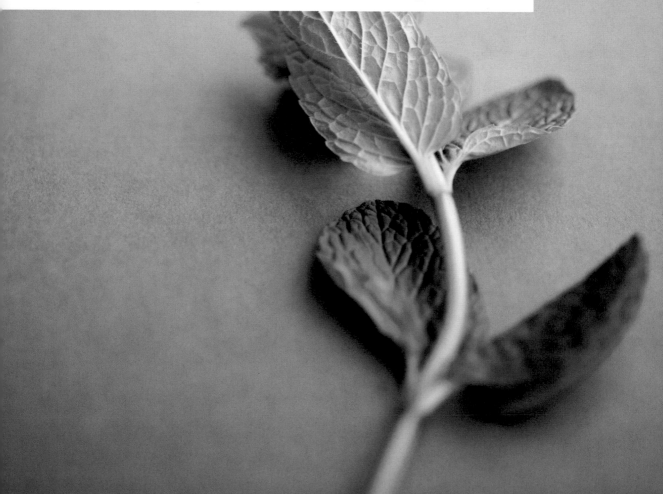

'We create habits and then our habits create us: STOP the habit that hurts us, KEEP the habit that supports us and START the habit that will make us grow.'

The stressed-out monk

Just as you can become fatigued by physical stress, your mental energy can become depleted by mental stress. Stressing out your inner Warrior Monk makes the stress hormone cortisol soar, and shuts down your body's fat-burning system. If those elevated stress levels go unchecked, high cortisol levels can result in weight gain, type-2 diabetes, high blood pressure and coronary artery disease. We all need to spend more time in the Zen garden!

MOOD FOOD

If you're feeling stressed: Spice up your mood with chilli – it'll spark the production of endorphins and make you feel awesome!

If you're feeling depressed: The omega-3 fatty acids found in fish will help pump up your mood. Splurge on salmon, tuna, mackerel or sardines at least once a week.

Feeling lethargic: You can feel deflated and lacking energy if you are low on iron. Get carnivore and hoe into some red meat. If you're vegie, binge on greens to unleash your inner warrior once again.

Monks that stress more

When it comes to what we eat and drink, there are three main culprits that get our inner warrior monks all stressed out:

1. **Faux food:** Processed foods and drinks, particularly those containing refined sugars, sodium and processed grains, cause higher insulin levels that trigger elevated cortisol levels and shut down the body's fat-burning system.

2. **Salt punch:** Sodium aids the conversion of cortisol in the body. Keep your salt intake to a minimum, preferably no more than 6 grams a day. You do need some iodised salt for thyroid support, but there is way too much sodium in processed foods for our inner monk to metabolise.

3. **Stresstails:** Drinking alcohol also increases those pernicious stress hormone levels in your body.

SHAOLIN MONK move

EAT NAKED

Eating healthily is the best way to transform negative thinking into positive thoughts, protect new brain cells and improve your mood. You need to do two things. Eat naked. And don't eat too much. Remember: there's no such thing as a bad food, only bad portions.

TIFFINY'S
EPIPHANY

The enemy of good mental health is stress. Mental stress is making us fat and unhappy, but the effects of stress are reversible.

Monks that stress less

De-stress your inner Warrior Monk with this fab four:

1. **High-five fibre:** Eat foods that are high in soluble fibre, like oat bran, oatmeal, beans, barley, apples and pears. Foods high in insoluble fibre are also the go, including wholewheat breads, wheat cereals, carrots and cooked cruciferous vegetables like cabbage, brussels sprouts and broccoli.

2. **Phosphatidylserine:** *Phospho* what? It's a natural chemical that buffers overproduction of cortisol in response to physical stress. Great sources of phosphatidylserine are mackerel, herring, eel, tuna, chicken, beans, beef, pork, whole grains, green leafy vegies and brown rice.

3. **Try tryptophan:** Tryptophan is an amino acid that increases serotonin, lowers cortisol and enhances your ability to deal with stress. Great sources of tryptophan are turkey meat, egg whites, spinach and crab.

4. **Vitamin C:** Plant sterols and vitamin C have been shown to inhibit cortisol levels during times of physical stress. Green vegetables and every kind of fruit can calm your inner monk. The best sources of vitamin C are citrus fruits, tomatoes, broccoli, turnips, sweet potatoes and cantaloupe. If it's bright orange, you'll get a vitamin C hit!

Insulin resistance

Stress caused by insulin resistance might be one reason why you reach for junk foods and feel depressed and tired. You can reduce insulin resistance by cooking with vinegar – it will slow the spike in your blood sugar levels. Why? Because the acetic acid in vinegar slows the rate at which your stomach empties.

Mix vinegar with olive oil for a healthy salad dressing or sprinkle some vinegar on your morning eggs. Another tip is to spice up your meals with a teaspoon of cinnamon on oats, in teas, on toast or as an extract to enhance insulin function and reduce blood sugar. Oh, and did I mention that exercise lowers blood sugar levels?

Metabolism yoga

When the stress hormone is stimulated, fat burn shuts down. Not fair! Try these tips to relax and restore your energy centre.

1. **Balance your hormones:** If you are suffering from stress, anxiety or insomnia, eat toxin free. Eliminate stress from your body by detoxing from soft drinks; avoid the trans fats found in most fried foods, baked goods and processed foods; give up alcohol and drugs; and steer clear of pesticides.

MONK MOMENT: BRAIN BINGE

Stress increases hunger. Bummer! Your body freaks when it loses energy through stress, and will send you out to hunt and gather in the pantry.

When the body is under stress, in fight-or-flight mode, sugar is retained in the bloodstream for easy access to energy. During prolonged periods of stress, high cortisol levels will continue to elevate your blood sugar levels and your hunger. So when you binge, it isn't because you are undisciplined, it's because you can't fight your body's natural instinct to physiologically fight stress by *finding food immediately*!

2. **Stretch out your energy levels:** Limit your intake of caffeine to one or two coffees a day. Or swap to some less hard-core teas like green, chamomile or dandelion.

3. **Purify your system:** Lose those artificial sweeteners – they're 300 times as sweet as sugar, and will only increase your cravings for sweetness.

    In fact, artificial sweeteners are such a no-no, the health industry is now heralding natural sugar as the new 'health food'. Try a natural sweetener like stevia, or use honey instead.

4. **Cleanse your metabolism:** Pile your plate high with curative foods like cabbage, broccoli, cauliflower, bok choy, brussels sprouts, asparagus and capsicum.

5. **Boost your antioxidants:** Detox your body by munching on **beans** – red kidney beans, black beans, pinto beans; **fruit** – blueberries, cranberries, blackberries, strawberries, apples; **vegies** – dark leafy greens; **nuts** – pecans, walnuts, hazelnuts; and **herbs 'n' spices** – cloves, cinnamon, oregano, dill, parsley.

Monk meditations on self-esteem

- Shift the energy of thinking about yourself to thinking about others. As my mum says: 'When you feel nervous, concentrate on service.' Much healthier!

- When you are suffering from low self-esteem, try not to think about how your body *looks* but how your body *feels*. If you *feel* healthy, then that's a win!

- Don't make happiness depend on happenstance: 'I'll be happy when ...' Forget tomorrow: joy is happiness that is independent of what happens to us in the future. It's all about being in the present. Good luck can make us happy, but it can't give us lasting joy.

- You are a superstar! Make an Oscar thank you speech in the mirror for winning the Best Human Being Award. List all your blessings and thank all the people who have helped you on your journey. If doing this does nothing more than make you laugh, then it's worth it.

Accept your inner monk

Stress often stems from thinking about what other people think of you. Building self-esteem is all about resilience: you can't control what others say or think of you, but you *can* control your opinion of yourself. When you are healthy in mind, body and spirit, you are rewarded with self-confidence.

COMBAT THREE TYPES OF STRESS BY EATING NAKED

Oxidative stress
This is stress at a cellular level – you can't see it, but the consequences can include lack of energy – the very energy that can help put a stop to that stress cycle. Eating naked reduces oxidative stress.

Blood sugar deregulation
Loading up on sugar and refined carbohydrates strains the hormones involved, as well as the cells' capacity to process sugar. The result: it further erodes your body's ability to produce energy, and sends the signal to keep the stress hormones coming. Eat naked and you reduce your intake of baddies like sugar and refined carbs.

Inflammation
Inflammation is caused by oxidative stress and blood sugar deregulation. It creates harmful chemicals that cause damage to important tissues, perpetuating a number of diseases including heart disease, depression and anxiety. Stripping your food of processing by eating naked reduces inflammation throughout the body.

Years ago, my sister gave me the best advice for dealing with my lack of confidence and fear of what other people thought of me: 'Everyone is too busy thinking about themselves to think about you. Do your best.' Once I realised that everyone was in fact too busy with their own stuff to give a second thought to my imperfections, I felt more confident.

Never feel embarrassed or ashamed. Everyone is dealing with stress in their lives.

Having **compassion** for others is **transforming**, because it replaces an unhealthy focus on the self.

TIFFINY'S
EPIPHANY

Get into your Mind Gym
with your inner Monk
Warrior to create new
thinking patterns and
positive thoughts.

Mentalaxation

Listen to your inner Shaolin monk when you're trying to lose weight and de-stress, and they'll tell you to control the inside first, the outside next. There is no point in stressing over things that are out of your control, outside of your body. Self-control works from the inside out. You can't control when you receive an email, how people will act, the weather, but you do have control over your body. Breathing reminds us of this …

FIVE BREATH MENTALAXATION

Focus your awareness on your breath for five full cycles. You can do this any time – at the beginning of a meal, when you're stopped in traffic or waiting in a line – and after a bit of practice it will work as a trigger. Whenever you begin to feel stressed out, anxious, angry, impatient – turn your attention towards your breathing. It will release those things around you that are out of your control and centre your mind on what you *can* control – your feelings. Five breaths may be all it takes to bring you back to awareness of yourself and put stress into perspective.

Monk magic

A healthy body grows from a healthy mind. In order to stop overeating because of stress, you need to be balanced in every aspect of your body.

CREATING A RESILIENT AND BALANCED BODY WITH MONK MAGIC

TYPE OF RESILIENCE	MONK MAGIC SOLUTION
Balance your brain chemistry	Diet, supplements, medications if needed
Manage your energy levels	Exercise, physical activities
Align yourself with nature's rhythms	Good sleep patterns, balanced hormones, regular cycles of activity and rest, a balanced lifestyle (health, relationships, self-development, wealth mastery and leisure)
Skilfully face emotions	Awareness of your inner experience, grounding you in the moment
Quieten the mind	Mindfulness of breath, thoughts and speech
Create deep connections	Open yourself up to self-acceptance through love, generosity and connection to others

WAVE YOUR WHITE FLAG
Don't be so hard on yourself.
When you're pregnant, you
need to surrender. You'll have
an uncontrolled urge to sleep.
So wave your white flag and
sleep. Remember that you
can't fight tiredness with food.

Approach motherhood as a monk not a martyr

Put those guilt bags down! Yes – I'm talking to you, Warrior Mums! You shouldn't feel guilty for wanting to be more healthy and take time out to exercise, lose weight and eat well. Prioritising your health journey is an integral part of self-acceptance, and a healthy mum means a healthier family. If you're not a Health Ninja Mum, you won't have healthy little ninjas!

You deserve to be a healthy warrior mother, so get ya ninja on! Put yourself first.

Eating for two

Pregnancy can be a great excuse to let yourself go by 'eating for two', or to overeat bad stuff while making the excuse of having cravings. Pregnancy is perhaps the most important time in your life to eat well and exercise regularly – after all, it's your nutrition that's developing your child.

Hormones go crazy when you are pregnant and there will be times when you would kill for some grease or sugar. Cravings will happen, but remember that old saying: you are what your mother eats. If you can stick to the 80 per cent Stoic Samurai, 20 per cent Naughty Ninja rule – that's pretty good!

MONK MOVE: MATERNAL MASTER

You may not have the energy and stamina to go to the supermarket, buy fresh fish and grill it with steamed vegies so you get the perfect weight loss meal. Who cares! If you choose water over another coffee, then that's a win. If you lie down for a 20-minute power nap with bub, that's a win! You are on the right track. Now's the time for you to be a Maternal Master: that means nurturing both your child and your inner self. And your partner – we mustn't forget about them!

Lose it, baby!

So many mothers come to me for advice on how they can lose their baby weight. Your best self-defence against baby weight gain begins before conception. If you are contemplating pregnancy, then aim to be at your optimal weight with a healthy BMI of between 25 and 30. If you fall pregnant when you're overweight, you're more likely to gain weight during your pregnancy and then have trouble losing it after your baby's birth. Being overweight can increase your long-term risk of diabetes, heart disease and some cancers – not good!

TIFFINY'S
EPIPHANY

You need to look after
yourself if you are to care for
your baby. Be gentle with yourself,
compassionate. Your body has just
done the most amazing stuff!
Honour yourself for that, and
break down your recovery
into baby steps.

If you are planning another pregnancy, it is a good idea to return to your pre-pregnancy weight before you conceive, or at least close to it. Starting your pregnancy at a BMI above the healthy weight range puts you and your baby at greater health risks during your pregnancy, and retaining excess weight over subsequent pregnancies increases your risk of lifestyle diseases.

Women who are overweight or who gain too much weight during pregnancy also have a higher risk of:

- High blood pressure
- Gestational diabetes during pregnancy
- Giving birth to a large baby
- Caesarean section
- Birth defects

HOW MUCH IS HEALTHY?

A healthy weight gain during pregnancy varies between individuals, but floats between 10 kilos and 15 kilos.

First trimester:
All women can expect to gain 1 or 2 kg in the first three months of pregnancy.

Second and third trimesters:
You should aim to gain:
BMI less than 18.5 = 500 g per week
BMI 18.5 to 24.9 = 400 g per week
BMI over 25 = less than 300 g per week

Having twins or triplets:
You will need to gain more weight over the course of your pregnancy:
BMI 18.5 to 24.9 = 16 to 24 kg
BMI 25 to 29.9 = 14 to 23 kg
BMI above 30 = 11 to 19 kg

Move it, baby!

It's important for Maternal Masters to stay active – don't be afraid to exercise during your pregnancy. You should do everything you did before you were pregnant – just not as intensely. A good guideline is the 'talk test' – while exercising, you should be able to easily hold a conversation without being short of breath.

Many activities are safe during pregnancy, including:

- Swimming
- Walking
- Cycling on an exercise bike
- Yoga or Pilates
- Low-impact aerobics, like water aerobics
- Light weights
- Non-contact martial arts
- Walk, walk, walk – before and after you have the baby

Baby classes

Classes that specially cater to pregnant women may be more suited to your needs and body changes during your pregnancy. The trainer can adapt the exercises for you, such as having you lie on your side rather than on your back.

Most activities are safe, as long as you:

- Take things easy
- Stop when you are tired
- Drink plenty of water
- Wear suitable clothing
- Don't become overheated
- Stop if you experience any pain
- Allow yourself recovery time after your exercise sessions – this may be two hours or two days. Listen to your body.

Exercises to avoid

- Excessive stretching – your ligaments will be softened by the hormonal changes you experience during pregnancy
- Avoid sidekicks in aqua aerobics and swimming breaststroke.
- Save sit-up type exercises until after your baby arrives – be conscious of any strain on your stomach muscles and your growing baby
- High-impact activities or contact sports – running, surfing, waterskiing, netball, football, contact martial arts or squash
- Activities that may limit your oxygen supply – scuba diving and mountain climbing, for example

TIFFINY'S EPIPHANY

When you walk, enjoy being outside surrounded by nature to enhance your feelings of wellbeing. Your good mood will affect your baby's mood.

BENEFITS OF EXERCISE DURING PREGNANCY

- Decreased lower back pain
- Less nausea
- Less heartburn
- Lower stress levels
- More energy
- Better bowel habits
- Better sleep patterns
- Lowered stress levels
- Less anxiety
- Lower risk of diabetes and heart disease
- Quicker return to normal after childbirth

- If you need help, lean on the people around you to provide assistance.
- Ask your parents or partner to make healthy snacks you can eat while rocking your baby.
- Set an alarm on your phone so you eat regularly.
- Don't allow sleep deprivation to rob you of sustenance.
- Join a mothers group – it will be a font of sanity, and you can talk about the things you're experiencing with other mothers who are feeling just like you.
- Rally a pram brigade to walk together.
- Attend postnatal classes.
- Split the cost of a trainer who specialises in postnatal exercise with your friends.
- Take your time, enjoy being maternal to your child and to yourself.

There's no such thing as 'bouncing back'

The greatest amount of weight loss occurs in the first three months after the birth of your child. Weight loss then continues at a slow and steady rate until six months after the birth. Breastfeeding can help you to return to your pre-pregnancy weight, as some of the weight you gained during your pregnancy is used as fuel to create breast milk. You can burn up 2500 kJ a day breastfeeding – that's nearly a whole block of chocolate every day – and that's why it's so important not to be underweight before conception.

But let's not push breastfeeding as a weight-loss weapon. Many women find it hard to establish successful breastfeeding patterns – it might be due to having had a Caesarean delivery, a complicated pregnancy or multiple births.

There's so much pressure for women to bounce back after the birth, what with celeb mums with nothing bigger than their new baby-feeding boobs. Well, those svelte mums on magazine covers can probably afford a nanny, private trainer, nutritionist, chef, stylist, PA and house staff to do all the stuff that stops you from getting out to exercise or having the time to cook yourself a healthy meal. When bub comes along, perhaps the only energy you have left after many sleepless nights is to make yourself a piece of toast and put some butter on it!

Pregnancy and giving birth isn't like having the flu – you don't bounce back. Forget that! You should never think about losing baby weight as 'bouncing back' but rather as recovery. You have surrendered your body for nine months to your gorgeous child. You have eaten what you felt your baby needed and let it grow, stretch and feed off you. No wonder you are tired and feeling a little depleted! If it took nine months to put the weight on, it will take at least eighteen months to lose it.

Losing baby weight should be looked at as a two-year recovery program. Something you slowly map and achieve in inch pebbles, not milestones. Approach your health the Three Hour Day way: make good decisions for yourself and your child every three hours, and if you slip-up, start again in three hours' time.

Ninja mums are tough mums

- Be organised with meal plans and healthy eating. When buggerlugs arrives you will be super busy, so plan ahead now: adopt healthy habits, rhythms of eating and build up a repertoire of quick, healthy, easy recipes that you'll be able to eat on the run.
- Indulge in some on-line supermarket shopping and home deliveries during the first few weeks to help with meal planning and to lighten the load.
- Use a baby monitor and during one of your baby's daytime sleeps, do some exercise at home – have fun with a Wii, a stationary bike, yoga, skipping rope. Not every day but two or three times a week.
- If you're breastfeeding, start expressing milk early on and freeze it to share the load and have time out.

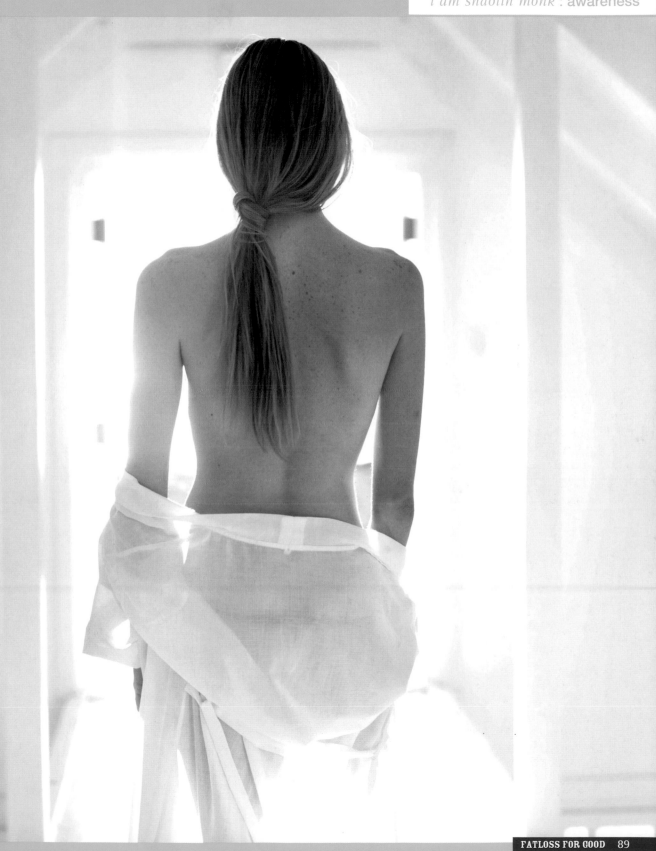

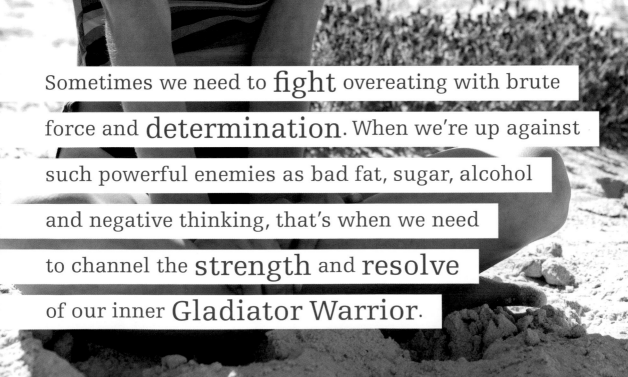

Sometimes we need to **fight** overeating with brute force and **determination**. When we're up against such powerful enemies as bad fat, sugar, alcohol and negative thinking, that's when we need to channel the **strength** and **resolve** of our inner **Gladiator Warrior**.

4

Love your **hunger**

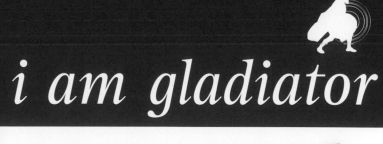

i am gladiator

strength

gladiator move

Food addiction makes you feel like you have to act on the compulsion to eat, but remember: thoughts aren't real. Boredom and frustration can make you *think* you are hungry, even when you're not. Ask yourself: am I really hungry or am I *emotionally* hungry?

Hunger hangover

Hunger has a bad reputation. We think of it as our enemy if we're on a diet, our ruin if we're caught up in a food frenzy. We live in a society that teaches us that hunger is something to be conquered, but in fact hunger isn't our foe, it's our friend.

My contestants on *The Biggest Loser* admitted they'd never ever known the feeling of hunger. Never! A huge challenge for me was teaching them to get to know their appetites and hunger cues. I taught them not to be afraid of hunger.

It's okay to feel hungry, it really is! Learn to listen to your body, and actually *feel* whether you are hungry, and you will learn to eat mindfully with the help of your inner gladiator. When we don't eat mindfully we make bad choices for our health – it's when junk food and hunger become the enemies we need to vanquish.

Eat only when you are hungry, and your body will tell you when it wants food – your stomach will bark. Wait for it, and learn to recognise your body's cues. When your stomach growls every four hours, it's a sign that your metabolism is speeding up. This is a really healthy sign.

Sometimes we can't fight binge eating with stealth like the ninja, with honour like the samurai or with the power of our minds like a Shaolin monk. Sometimes it takes a gladiator! Learning to deal with hunger will set you free from the fear of feeling hungry and the consequences of that fear: overeating. Hunger will trigger your natural gladiator instincts, and stop you being a slave to constant feeding. Learn to love your hunger!

APPETITE CONTROL

It's true: you *can* tolerate feeling a little hungry, so get to work on your appetite control. A mild level of hunger will improve your concentration and keep your mind sharp. After a while, you may recognise that what once felt like starvation is actually just a little mid-morning digestion. As you become attuned to your hunger, your stomach will adapt and shrink. Your brain chemistry will regulate the 'full' and 'hungry' hormones, and telegraph the correct appetite cues.

Hunger games

To win the hunger games, your inner gladiator needs to learn how to distinguish the hunger grand final from the emotional play-offs. The two codes play by completely different rules.

'Always ask the question:

am I really hungry or am I

emotionally hungry?'

gLaᴅɪatoʀ move
TIME TO EAT

Tick-tock, it's 12 o'clock. Are you feeling hungry? Perhaps not. If you are truly feeling hungry, then by all means have your lunch. However, if you're not, go for a walk instead and eat later on, when you really are hungry.

Emotional play-offs
- The desire to eat arises from thoughts, feelings or situations rather than physical hunger
- The feeling comes on suddenly and involves cravings for a certain type of food
- The feeling leads to mindless munching or unconscious eating
- Emotional hunger often ends in eating beyond the point of satisfaction, followed by feelings of guilt

Hunger grand final
- A feeling of hunger occurs naturally every 3-4 hours, with symptoms of a growling stomach, a sensation of emptiness and perhaps a slight headache, fatigue and dizziness
- The feeling is gradual, and can be satiated by a variety of foods
- The feeling leads to an increasing awareness of food choices and portions
- Eating mindfully means eating until physically satisfied, with no associated guilt
- You feel refuelled and ready to go.

Not hungry but hurting with emotional hunger
Get yourself some sleep, if you can – the world is a different place when you wake up. Then blow off some steam by:
- Listening to some relaxing music
- Going for a walk
- Seeing a movie
- Meeting up with a friend
- Taking 10 deep breaths or practising meditation
- Enjoying a bubble bath
- Buying someone you love a gift

Dining-out wars
The good news is that dining out with family and friends at restaurants and fast-food joints is fine if you're trying to shed a few extra kilos. By using visual cues to create properly portioned meals, and by paying attention to the wording of menu items, you can continue to lose weight while dining out and still savour many of your favourite dishes – even dessert. The key is to be **pro portion** and to make wise menu choices.

DINING-OUT DOGMA

Read menus carefully, and select items that are high in flavour but low in kilojoules and fat. The general rule is to go for dishes that are steamed, baked or grilled, and pass on anything cheesy, creamy or fried. Choose a salad with low-fat dressing or fresh vegetables without butter or oil, and you can just about eat as much as you like.

Portion precaution

The most important factor when dining out is portion size. The size of an average restaurant meal has doubled in the past 25 years, so be sure to modify your choices accordingly:

- Choose a low-fat starter and a side salad instead of ordering a main meal
- Share a main meal with a friend
- Order one dessert for everyone to share, or choose a fresh fruit salad or sorbet
- Dine by choice not by chance – choose a restaurant in advance, then go online to preview the menu and make your selection before you arrive
- Know what serving size is appropriate for you

Decoding the menu

Keep your gladiator wits about you when you're browsing the menu – it's bound to be full of traps for the unwary:

- Beware the preparation spin: avoid anything labelled 'secret sauce' and words like 'smothered', 'old-fashioned' and 'meaty'.
- Beware of code words for HUGE: supreme, king-size, double, jumbo, super-sized, whopper, club, deluxe, the works, ultimate, triple-decker. These menu items will most likely be two or even three times larger than the regular portion size.
- Recognise those fat cues: deep-fried, golden, crispy, crunchy, crumbed, creamed, fritter, breaded, battered, buttered, roasted, crusted, sautéed, stuffed, aioli, gratin, beurre, bisque, carbonara, Alfredo, tempura, béchamel.
- Choose dishes with 'good' words: baked, barbecued, boiled, braised, broiled, broth, coulis, garden fresh, grilled, poached, raw, roasted, salsa, steamed.

TIFFINY'S EPIPHANY

Remember to keep serves in proportion: big portions are worse than bad food.

TIFFINY'S EPIPHANY

Sometimes we panic when we feel hungry, but I want you to sit with it for a while, say for at least 20 minutes. You should only eat when you feel hungry and your body is asking for food. Wait for your body to ask for food before you feed it. Ask yourself, have I ever *really* felt ravenous? If the answer is no, you need to experience this feeling in order to understand your appetite cues.

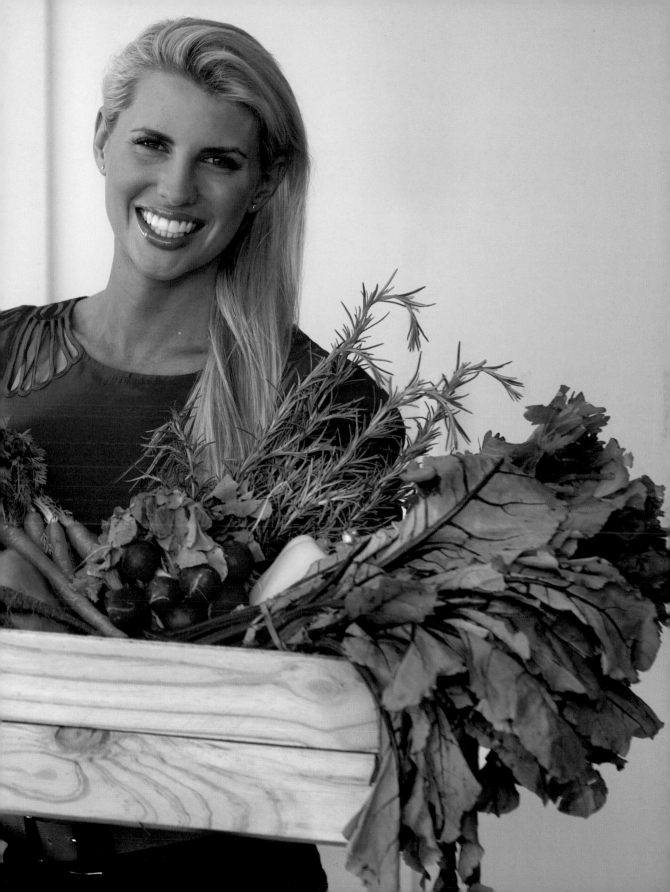

Restaurant tips

Get ya gladiator on when you're entering the arena of temptation:

- Don't order soft drinks or alcohol to drink with your meal – stick to an appetite suppressant, not an appetite stimulant, and fill up with water.
- Ask the waiter not to bring the bread basket to your table.
- Order first: you'll be less influenced by food envy – other people's choices.
- Ask for all sauces and dressings to be served on the side.
- Ask if you can have a salad instead of creamy or fried vegetables with your meal.
- Ask if you can substitute balsamic vinegar for mayonnaise or salad dressing.

WHEN YOU'RE DINING OUT, REMEMBER THESE PORTION GUIDELINES:

Meat = a deck of cards or the size of your fist
Fish = the size of a chequebook
Pasta and casseroles = enough to fill a quarter of your plate
Use a smaller plate – the bigger the bowl, the more you'll eat
Smaller utensils = smaller bites

Takeaway tips

Gladiators never deprive themselves of a treat now and then, but before you grab the plastic cutlery and chopsticks, consider these tips:

- **Sushi:** Stick to sashimi, and order your favourite combos as hand rolls with no rice. You can do this with almost any type of roll. Remember: often the white rice in sushi rolls is sweetened with sugar, so exercise pro portion.
- **Chinese:** Choose a dish that isn't breaded and deep-fried (goodbye, egg rolls!). Avoid rice and noodles, and steer clear of sugary sauces like sweet and sour. Opt for dishes that pair meat with a vegetable and serve the sauce on the side; for instance, beef and broccoli, shrimp and snow peas.
- **Thai:** Any of the satay dishes are delicious and nutritious – chicken, shrimp, beef or a vegetable stir-fry. Or go for steamed fish, chicken or beef lettuce rolls. Avoid fatty coconut-milk curries or noodle and rice dishes.
- **Indian:** The best bets include chicken, lamb, beef or shrimp *tikka* – grilled marinated meat skewers, in other words. Vegie dishes such as *bhagan bharta* (whipped eggplant), *saag paneer* (spinach with cottage cheese), *aloo gobi* (marinated steamed cauliflower and potatoes) and *jalfrezi* (mixed vegetables) are fine. Avoid curries, rice and naan bread.

Toxic takeaway for kids

Here's something that will make you think twice before ordering that burger or pizza for your family. Yale University's Rudd Centre analysed the calories, fat, sugar and sodium contained in more than 3000 items marketed as kids' meals. They then ranked them 'best' and 'worst' based on the guidelines that preschool children should consume no more than 410 calories (1712 kJ) and 544 milligrams of sodium per meal.

And you know what? Only a measly 1 per cent of the kids' meal combos qualified as 'best'. The vast majority weren't ranked at all, since they were all 'equally bad'. Here are some of the best and worst kids' meal combinations served at four popular fast-food chains:

TIFFINY'S EPIPHANY

If you're dining out late, eat a healthy snack beforehand so you don't arrive starving and go hoeing into the bread basket.

CHOOSE WISELY

Subway
Best: Vegie Delite Sandwich (wheat bread, no cheese)
- Calories: 205 (856 kJ)
- Sodium: 285 mg
- Fat: 0.9 g

Worst: Six-inch Meatball Sub
- Calories: 465 (1941 kJ)
- Sodium: 1200 mg
- Fat: 19.9 g

Hungry Jacks
Best: Garden salad with grilled chicken and French dressing
- Calories: 197 (822 kJ)
- Sodium: 055 mg
- Fat: 2.4 g

Worst: Ultimate Double Whopper
- Calories: 1277 (5331 kJ)
- Sodium: 2247 mg
- Fat: 83.9 g

KFC
Best: Original Burger
- Calories: 431 (1799 kJ)
- Sodium: 969 mg
- Fat: 14.5 g

Worst: Wicked Wings
- Calories: 1380 (5726 kJ)
- Salt: 2497 mg
- Fat: 02.3 g

McDonald's
Best: Seared chicken tandoori wrap
- Calories: 319 (1332 kJ)
- Sodium: 596 mg
- Fat total: 7.5 g

Worst: Double Quarter Pounder
- Calories: 853 (3561 kJ)
- Sodium: 1690 mg
- Fat: 53.4 g

Domino's Pizza
Best: Penne pasta with roasted chicken, mushrooms and tomato
- Calories: 387 (1616 kJ)
- Sodium: 575 mg
- Fat: 1.7 g

Worst: Meatlovers traditional puff pizza
- Calories per slice: 298 (1214 kJ)
- Sodium per slice: 716 mg
- Fat per slice: 16.7 g

Your body is always trying to stay balanced. When you binge on sugar, your body craves salty foods to rebalance and restore equilibrium. Think about your big nights out: booze (sugar) doesn't usually come with a salad, but a kebab (salt) or chips (fat). See? If you have Thai food (salt), within 30 minutes you're craving chocolate (sugar). It's not you, it's the chemistry of craving.

Gallivanting gladiators

When you're travelling on holidays, you don't have to let healthy eating and exercise fly out the window. Keeping on track while you're on the road (or on a cruise ship or in a plane) isn't as hard as it seems.

- Bring along an empty water bottle when you're catching a plane. You may not be allowed to take liquids through security, but you can fill up your water bottle at a drinking fountain once you pass through the checkpoint. It's vital to keep hydrated when you're flying, and if you're thirsty you'll crave more food. Your body is more sensitive to hunger than thirst, and that airplane food is packed with sodium, leaving you feeling even more thirsty!
- Ditch alcohol on flights. Flying already dehydrates you, and the booze will leave you feeling parched and asking for pretzels.
- Pack an in-flight lunchbox of healthy goodies to nibble – the trays of food they hand out on long-haul international flights are packed with calories! Try this for an eight-hour hour flight: a mix of raw nuts (include some licorice and a few squares of dark choc for the movies), 2 cans of tuna, 2 small cans of beans, green teabags, a couple of health bars, dry crackers, travel calm tablets, celery tablets and spirulina tablets. Celery tablets will help to reduce fluid retention caused from flying, while spirulina is a super supplement packed with a wide range of minerals, vitamins and phytonutrients to help combat jetlag and air sickness.
- Ask the airline about special meal options such as low-fat or vegetarian meals and pre-order them.
- Plan an active holiday, such as a walking tour instead of a bus tour, or a tennis camp instead of a cruise.
- Remember to pack your exercise clothes so you can walk, run and explore your new city, or work out in the hotel gym.

ɢʟᴀᴅɪᴀᴛᴏʀ move
STICKY-ICKY LAW

When fighting your sweet enemy, don't forget your inbuilt enemy detector – your tongue! If it tastes sweet – be suspicious, 'cos sticky can mean icky. Sticky drinks like juice, soft drinks and performance drinks have way too much sugar. Your tongue detector never lies!

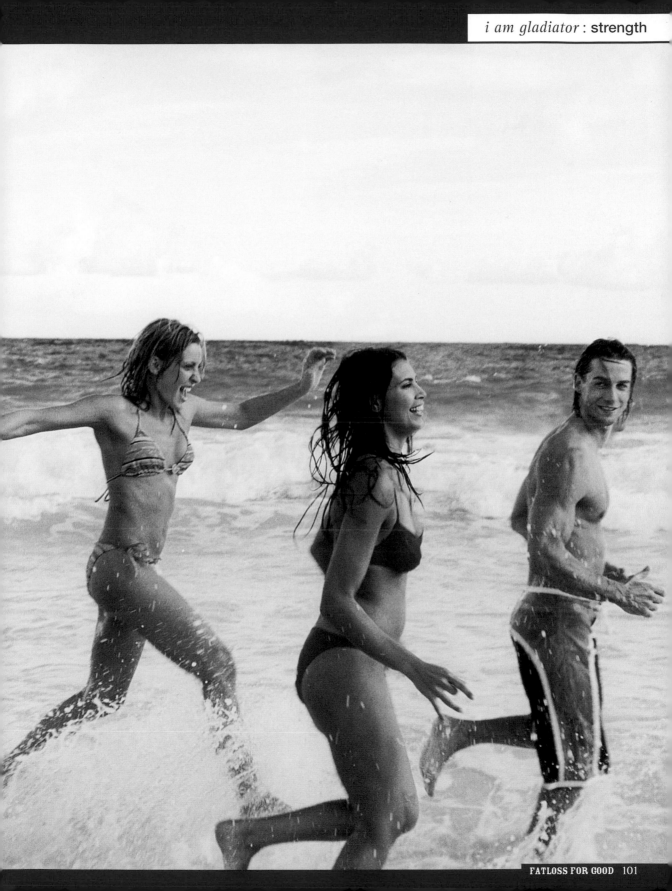

Gladiator teamwork

Maximise the nutritional kick of food by pairing ingredients with their famous partners.

- Strawberries and almonds aid the absorption of elegiac acid, famous for its cancer-fighting abilities.

- Tomatoes and olive oil are a classic combo. Tomatoes are packed with lycopene, a powerful fat-soluble antioxidant, and olive oil facilitates the body's absorption of it.

- Fish and lemon – lemon provides vitamin C, which promotes digestion by pumping up digestive enzymes. These help to break down fat and increase hydrochloric acid to help break down the fish, which is high in protein. Your body will absorb iron more effectively too. Winner!

- Onion and garlic enhance each other's potency as antioxidant, antibacterial and antiparasitic foods.

- Red meat and sage/greens – sage helps counteract the bad chemicals produced in charred or burnt meat. Your body soaks up more iron when meat is teamed with greens, which also helps digestion.

- Cashews and sunflower seeds are rich in calcium and magnesium. Eating them simultaneously means they are more likely to be bio-available to the body.

- Capsicum and spinach – foods high in vitamin C such as capsicum and iron-rich foods such as spinach help the body to absorb plant iron. Couples that fight together, stick together. If you are cooking these foods, the vitamin C in the capsicum will protect the folate in the spinach.

KILL CALORIES WITH A WORKOUT

Light exercise: walking, golf, housework, gardening, yoga
If you weigh 60 kg – you kill 3 calories (13 kJ) a minute
If you weigh 100 kg – you kill 5 calories (21 kJ) a minute

Moderate exercise: swimming, tennis, light weight-training, dancing
If you weigh 60 kg – you kill 5 calories (21 kJ) a minute
If you weigh 100 kg – you kill 7 calories (29 kJ) a minute

Heavy exercise: intense weight/resistance training, high heart rate running, martial arts
If you weigh 60 kg – you kill 8 calories (33 kJ) a minute
If you weigh 100 kg – you kill 12 calories (50 kJ) a minute

TIFFINY'S EPIPHANY

My foodosophy is simple when it comes to keeping myself in shape: move every day and eat whatever I like, in portions, as long as it ain't sweet.

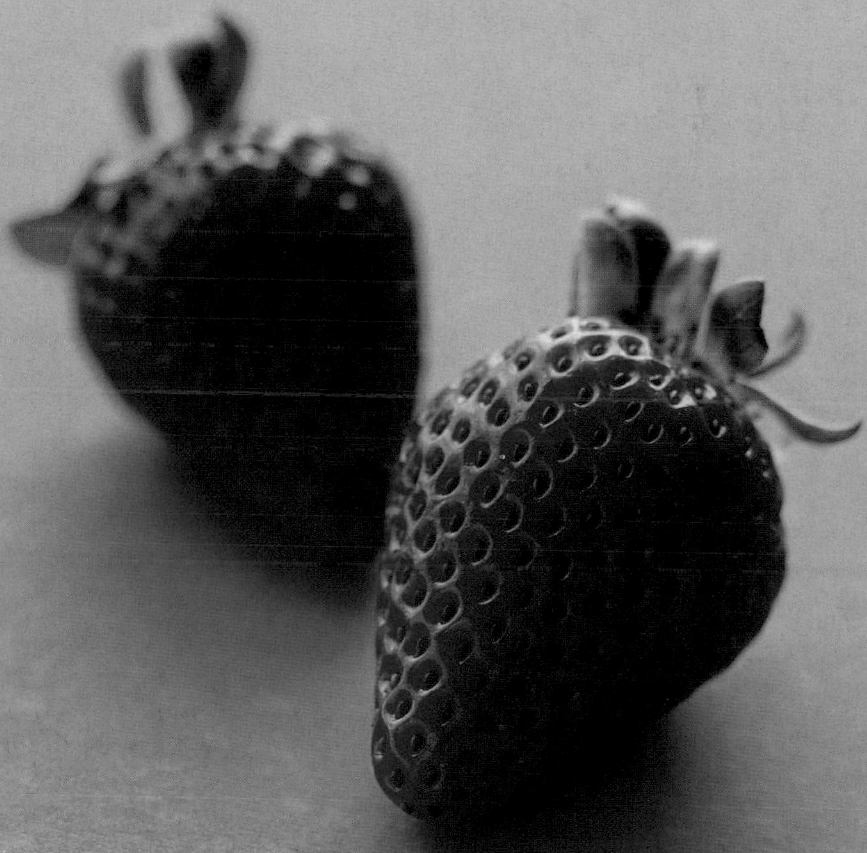

Always take the stairs – *always*! I can't remember the last time I took an elevator when travelling. Since it's more difficult to get my exercise when I'm away from my Health Gladiator equipment – namely my dojang, kick pads, bike and free weights – I get it every other way I can. And that means getting to know the stairwell. If you're staying on the 10th floor of your hotel, that's just great. You'll look better lying at the pool after you've been back and forth to your room a few times.

ɢʟᴀᴅɪᴀᴛᴏʀ move

Milk: 2 cups of skim milk or 1.5 cups of low-fat milk or equivalent soy/yoghurt/tofu drink.
Fat: Avoid as much trans fat and saturated fat as possible but fill up on good fats – at least 3 teaspoons of oil, 1.5 tablespoons of mayonnaise or half an avocado, 1.5 tablespoons of peanut butter or 30 g nuts and seeds.

- When in Rome – if the city you are visiting is famous for an activity, such as the tango in Buenos Aires, take a class.
- The best way to explore a new city is to walk it. Sure, you can save time riding a bus or subway, but just think how many calories you'll burn if you walk to all those museums and restaurants instead. Make it an adventure by getting hold of a map and scoping out a great route through the city's best sights.
- If you're near a beach, go paddleboarding, surfing or windsurfing. If you're near mountains, go for a bike ride or hike.
- To avoid vacation weight gain, start the day with a gigantic breakfast, followed by a light dinner. You'll save money too, as breakfast is always cheaper than dinner.
- McDonald's, KFC, Krispy Kreme – this junk food is everywhere, so why would you eat it on vacation?! Use your precious time on vacation to sample the local food. No Starbucks!

Corporate gladiators

Travelling on business? These simple suggestions will fit easily into even the busiest travel itineraries:

- If you're flying on a two-hour domestic flight, you don't have to eat in those two hours just because everyone else on board is snacking away. Attempt to fasten your mouth when you fasten your seatbelt on flights!
- Ask your employer to book you a vegetarian or low-fat meal.
- When the cabin crew drive by with their 'calorie carts', decline the tray and ask for water and a piece of fruit instead.
- Pack a few nonperishable, low-fat snacks to tide you over on the plane and in-between meetings. Check out the lunchbox recipes at the back of this book, or try raw nuts, vegetable sticks, tahini, muesli, rice cakes, homemade savoury muffins and fruit. Homemade trail mix is a winning plane snack: it's healthy, easy to carry and can be eaten a little at a time. Take a sturdy resealable bag and add your favourite nuts, such as cashews or almonds; two types of dried fruit, such as cranberries and goji berries;

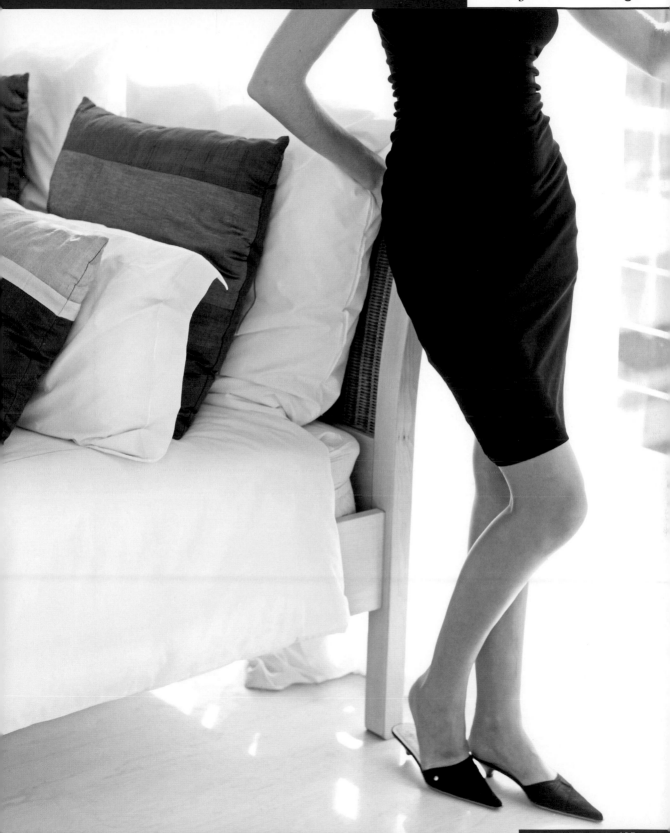

plus some pumpkin or sunflower seeds. Homemade snacks will divert you from airport fast food, dodgy muesli bars and – heaven help us – Pringles.

- Take advantage of the big buffet hotel breakfast. This will sustain you for seven hours, and you never know where your next meal may come from on a tight business schedule.
- If you get locked into a gazillion business lunches and dinners, choose your meal wisely – steamed vegies, grilled meats, fresh salads. **If you can't choose your meal, then choose your portion.** Try to skip dessert and alcoholic beverages.
- If your hotel doesn't have a gym, find some stairs. Go up and down as many flights as you can for a terrific workout.
- If you're feeling stressed, don't take it out on your minibar. Travel with passionflower herbal extract and St John's wort to relieve anxiety.

SUGAR STOP

Once you've stopped buying sugary products, stop the sugar spikes and crashes by eating protein at every meal. Protein promotes a feeling of fullness and will block any cravings. For backup, take a chromium mineral supplement to improve your blood sugar regulation and to help curb cravings.

Avoid the squirts – sauces, dressings and toppings are packed with sugar. Sweet chilli sauce has 10.4 g of sugar per tablespoon! Always opt for sugar-free sauces and dressings – vinegar, lemon and Tabasco are your mates.

Make sure to get breakfast in – not brunch! When you eat breakfast early in the day, you prevent the drop in blood sugar that makes you crave sweet things later on. Better still, eat a fat breakfast! A 'good fat' breakfast will keep you feeling full until lunchtime or even linner (early dinner). Try avocado and tomato on rye toast with cinnamon, an omelette with ham, or cottage cheese with shavings of nuts.

TIFFINY'S EPIPHANY

If you're an emotional eater, seek help first from a therapist, and then from a trainer. If you don't understand what's making you overeat, you'll never be able to lose weight long term. I'm as much a therapist on *The Biggest Loser* as I am a trainer. We work through stuff just as much as we work out.

15-MINUTE WORKOUT

If you're pressed for time with a busy agenda of meetings, squeeze in a 15-minute workout. Just 15 minutes will boost your metabolism all day, and clear your mind for your meetings. Warm up with any cardio activity for 5 minutes, then go hard for 2 minutes until you feel exhausted. Repeat this cycle twice, with a 30-second recovery, then finish with a heart-pumping 2 minutes of intense work and a cool down. You can do this by running on the spot, running up and down the hotel stairs, doing sprints outside, or a series of squat jumps, push-ups, jumping lunges and skipping in your room.

Best in-flight snacks

Virgin Blue
The best Virgin snacks are the banana bread slice and tasty cheese and crackers – both under 200 calories (835 kJ). Or skip the snacks and request a light meal such as the pumpkin soup or gluten-free noodle salad with requested gluten-free sauce. The roast beef sandwich is another good option, but avoid the ham and cheese wrap with mayonnaise – the mayo is packed with more calories than the wrap.

Qantas
Qantas are always good with the fresh fruit, so go for fruit over the dodgy muesli bars, salted nuts, muffin or biscuits. Qantas dinners are sauce-laden and sodium-packed: pack your own or skip it. Always go for the mesclun salad or grilled chicken over the penne pasta or rice and Asian greens. Give your bread roll to your neighbour.

Jetstar
Jetstar snacks are salty as – forget those cups of noodles, miso soup, savoury spicy broad beans, assorted nuts and Pringles, and stick with tasty cheese and crackers. Keep your bloat blinkers on for the oven-baked gourmet muffin, Byron Bay cookie bar, M&Ms and Mars Bar. The fresh sandwiches are spoiled with a lather of mayonnaise, but the gourmet chicken wrap will give you more protein and the mayo is less heavy.

Gladiator enemy #1: phantom fat
The reason Australia is the fattest country on the planet isn't because of fat, it's because of sugar.

Sugar is an appetite stimulant – I've seen it firsthand on *The Biggest Loser*. The contestants are always total sugar addicts – the more sugar they eat, the more they crave. But all sugars aren't the same. Glucose and fructose are both forms of sugar, but they're metabolised differently. Fructose is particularly dangerous 'cos it converts to body fat more quickly and shuts down our appetite hormones so we can't tell that we're full!

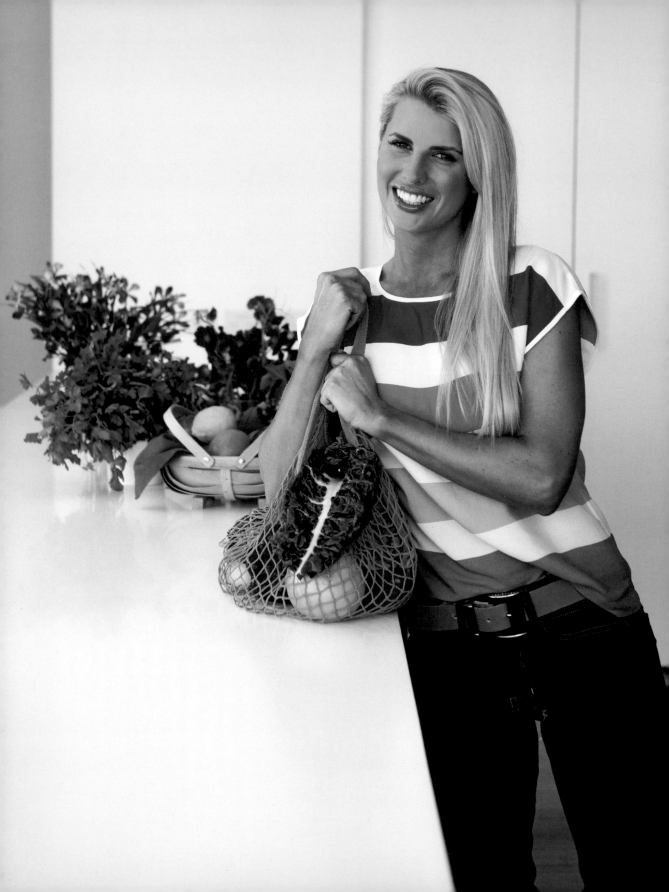

High-fructose foods include sultanas, fruit juices, leeks, onions, honey and wheat products. Apples, pears, watermelon and fruit juices are the most potent – I'm not saying fruit is bad for you, but if you bloat after eating these particular fruits, you may be fructose sensitive. Processed and fast foods are also high in fructans, including most beers, breads, cakes, biscuits, breakfast cereals, pies, pastas, pizzas and some noodles.

Foods containing sorbitol are also a problem and this includes some diet drinks, many chewing gums and sugar-free lollies. Xylitol is present in some sugar alcohols, such as erythritol, mannitol and other ingredients that end with -tol, commonly added as artificial sweeteners in processed foods.

The liver acts like a kind of traffic cop, sorting out whether the body needs to store glucose, burn it for energy or turn it into triglycerides, a type of fat found in the blood. But when fructose enters the body, it bypasses this process and ends up being quickly converted into body fat.

When we eat fat, the body has an appetite control to sense when we are full. But when it comes to sugar? Nope. No such control exists. Sugar is the ultimate stealthy enemy because it is completely invisible to your body. It's very high in calories but offers zero nutrition, so you get no bang for your calorie buck!

Just like a drug, sugar is addictive and the high is fleeting. And here's the not-so-sweet kicker: sugar messes up your metabolism and immune system, your teeth and the digits on the scales, and hands us a serve of type 2 diabetes. And when your sweet toxin has gone … you're left with crashing blood sugar levels and a body aching, craving, lusting for its next hit.

gladiator newsflash
LOW FAT STAT
'Low fat' doesn't mean 'low calories': a 'low-fat' apricot scroll from a bakery may have less than 2 grams of fat but it'll be stacked with a monstrous 415 calories because it is stuffed with 47.6 grams of sugar.

Sweet advice
First off, limit your intake of packaged foods that contain a lot of refined sugars – in other words, be wary of anything that isn't 'naked'. Food disguised in packaging can be crammed with surreptitious sugar – so you gotta strip it down!
- Read the label and watch out for sucrose, glucose, dextrose, fructose, maltose and HFCS. Alarm bells should ring for syrups, honeys and molasses, too.
- Combine your sugar with fibre by eating whole fruits.
- Better still, try combining whole fruits with good fats – try berries with nuts, or avocado on toast with honey. The good fats will slow down the absorption of sugar in your system.

Second, swap sugar for something else.
- Use the natural plant sweetener stevia in tea and coffee, on breakfast porridge and cereal, or in yoghurt.
- Banish liquid lollies (soft drinks!) – they're packed with sugar (some have more than 10 teaspoons of sugar per can) and additives.
- Squeeze fresh juices or dilute fruit juices with mineral water to make your own soft drinks.

- If you love juice but find it too sugary, try a smoothie: add natural yoghurt, nuts or LSA mix and rice milk.
- Keep jars of nuts, seeds and dried goji berries at the coffee station at work, by the kettle or in the pantry at home instead of biscuits – this way, when you have a snack attack while the kettle boils, you won't be tempted to splurge on sugar.
- Try using natural sweeteners when recipes call for sugar: stevia, date sugar made from ground dates, dried fruit, agave syrup, Manuka honey, molasses or pure maple syrup.

Third, block sugar from everyday use and read food labels carefully. Tomato ketchup can have up to 126 grams of sugar in a bottle, so think twice before going on the sauce! A bowl of Fruit Loops has more sugar in it than an entire packet of Tim Tams! Given the choice, I'd prefer the Tim Tams for breakfast, thanks!

- Steer clear of products that list sugar in the first three ingredients.
- Trash the junk food in your fridge and pantry and replace it with sugar-free snacks.
- Swap chocolate for carob or (low-sugar) health bars.
- Make savoury muffins, fruit slices and wholemeal cakes, and always bake with stevia instead of sugar.
- Snack on hummus and vegie sticks, rice crackers and natural peanut butter paste.
- Forget the breakfast cereal offenders laden with sugar and opt for whole oat porridge, quinoa, millet, buckwheat and natural muesli. Sweeten them with fresh or dried fruit, vanilla or cinnamon.
- Yoghurt can contain up to 20 grams of sugar, so watch for spiked sugar in your tubs – 'low-fat' doesn't mean 'low sugar'. Buy plain yoghurt and sweeten it yourself with puréed fruit, stevia, nuts, seeds or natural muesli.
- Forget sugar spreads like jam, marmalade and Nutella. Instead, try small amounts of prune or date spread, nut paste, a smashed avocado, banana or my favourite, unhulled tahini.

DON'T EAT AND DRIVE

If food flies in through the window of your car – it's not food! Your car isn't a kitchen or a restaurant. Eating unconsciously derails your health and fitness, and leads to overeating. Distract your mind and break the habit of eating and driving – listen to a book instead, or learn a language on CD. If you eat and drive, you will pack pounds.

Sugar snap guide

1 tsp = 5 g = 20 calories (89 kJ)
1 tbsp = 16 g = 65 calories (271 kJ)
Rectangular sachet = 1 tsp = 20 calories (89 kJ)
Coffee shop sugar stick = 3 g = 12 calories (50 kJ)
Coffee shop raw sugar stick = 3 g = 12 calories (50 kJ)
1 tbsp brown sugar = 16 g = 45 calories (183 kJ)
½ cup caster sugar = 450 calories (1879 kJ)
½ cup icing sugar = 285 calories (1190 kJ)
CSR 50% reduced sugar:
½ tsp = 2 g = 8 calories (33 kJ)
coffee shop sugar stick = 2 g = 8 calories (33 kJ)
1 sachet Equal = 2 tsp = 5 calories (21 kJ) (bar the chemicals, which are mind blowing!)
1 tsp stevia = 1 calorie (4 kJ)

gladiator newsflash

SUGAR SOUP

'Healthy' doesn't necessarily mean sugar free, especially when it comes to cereals – many breakfast foods are cereal killers with up to 30 per cent sugar! Anything more than 8 g sugar on any label is ludicrous – it's like eating sugar soup! Ditch that heavy bowl of sugar soup for breakfast and have mashed sweet potato with your eggs instead of cornflakes.

Gladiator enemy #2: stress fat

When we talk down to ourselves, criticise ourselves, berate and begrudge ourselves, we create stress. Get the emotions involved with those negative thoughts, and the body reciprocates with tightened muscles, headaches, dehydration, cramps – in a word, we fall apart!

Anxiety, depression and insomnia have all been associated with the production of excess insulin. Increased insulin also results from eating too much sugar and refined carbohydrates, and not moving enough, which in turn elevates inflammation and stress hormones. *Ah ha!* In addition, excess insulin deprives the brain of its steady supply of glucose for fuel, further heightening our state of anxiety.

Most of us have stress in our daily lives – we learn to live with it – but if your daily life is filled with constant, unremitting stress, it can be dangerous. What determines how well you handle chronic stress is how you respond to it and your ability to shut stress down and chill out. And wouldn't you know it, one of the most stressful things you can do to yourself is to go on a diet!

Gladiator fat factories

The equation is simple: every kilogram of muscle burns three times more calories than a kilo of fat. Muscles spoon up blood sugar and enhance your body's insulin sensitivity. The more muscle you have, the more cells are available to absorb glucose, and you don't have to produce as much insulin after eating. Your muscle cells are more efficient at using glucose for fuel, so your body doesn't have to store as much food as fat. Plus, every kilo of muscle burns up to 400 calories (1670 kJ) just to sustain itself. That's a free meal a day!

Gladiator move
MILK CHOCOLATE

I'm not saying ditch the chocolate – I'm not crazy! – but it's important to understand the amount of energy lurking in that little square of heaven. Calorie wise, a row is almost equal to an entire meal!

1 row (6 pieces) = 130 calories (543 kJ) (equivalent to 4 McDonalds chicken McNuggets)

2 rows = 265 calories (1106 kJ) (for this calorie price, you could have a whole cookies and cream cheesecake dessert from KFC)

If you want to lose weight, you have to hit specific nude food targets. **Buy a calorie counter and learn the energy value of food.** The more you weigh, the more energy you use in a day, so you'll need to consume a higher amount of calories. Similarly, the more you weigh, the more calories you will burn in a day:

- If you want to lose up to 5 kilos, females need to reach 1200 calories (5010 kJ), males 1600 calories (6680 kJ) – take in fewer calories, and you stimulate the body's starvation response
- If you want to lose 6-15 kilos, females need to hit 1500 calories (6263 kJ), males 1900 calories (7933 kJ)
- If you want to lose 26-50 kilos, females need to hit 1900 calories, (7933 kJ) males 2300 calories (9603 kJ)

Fatloss Warrior tips

1. Stay allergic to crash diets that make you fluctuate in weight. When you lose weight and then regain it, second-generation fat is more difficult to melt.
2. Control your insulin – eat whole carbs and stabilise your insulin by incorporating essential fatty acids into your diet such as salmon, mackerel, herring, walnuts, almonds, dark green vegies, olive oil, flaxseed oil, wholegrain foods, lean meats and eggs.
3. Minimise your grog intake.
4. Move it! A healthy diet and exercise are the best defence against stubborn fat. But don't overtrain. If you stress out your body with exercise, it will have the opposite effect and slow down your metabolism.
5. If food or water stinks of plastic, don't go near it. Compounds in plastic called plasticisers have been found to be highly carcinogenic. Plasticisers can leak into water, milk or foods that are packaged. Another reason to eat naked!

GOOD FATS

The human brain is 60% fat – so no wonder the body needs good fats:

- Fat maintains the nervous system, your brain's SMS communication with the rest of your body.
- Fat boosts your immune system and acts as a Gladiator shield to keep out dangerous germs and microbes that can cause illness.
- Fat is needed by all the cells in your body: nerve cells, eye cells, brain cells and even heart cells need fat to survive.
- Your body needs fat in order to properly absorb and use crucial vitamins such as A, D, E, K and beta-carotene.

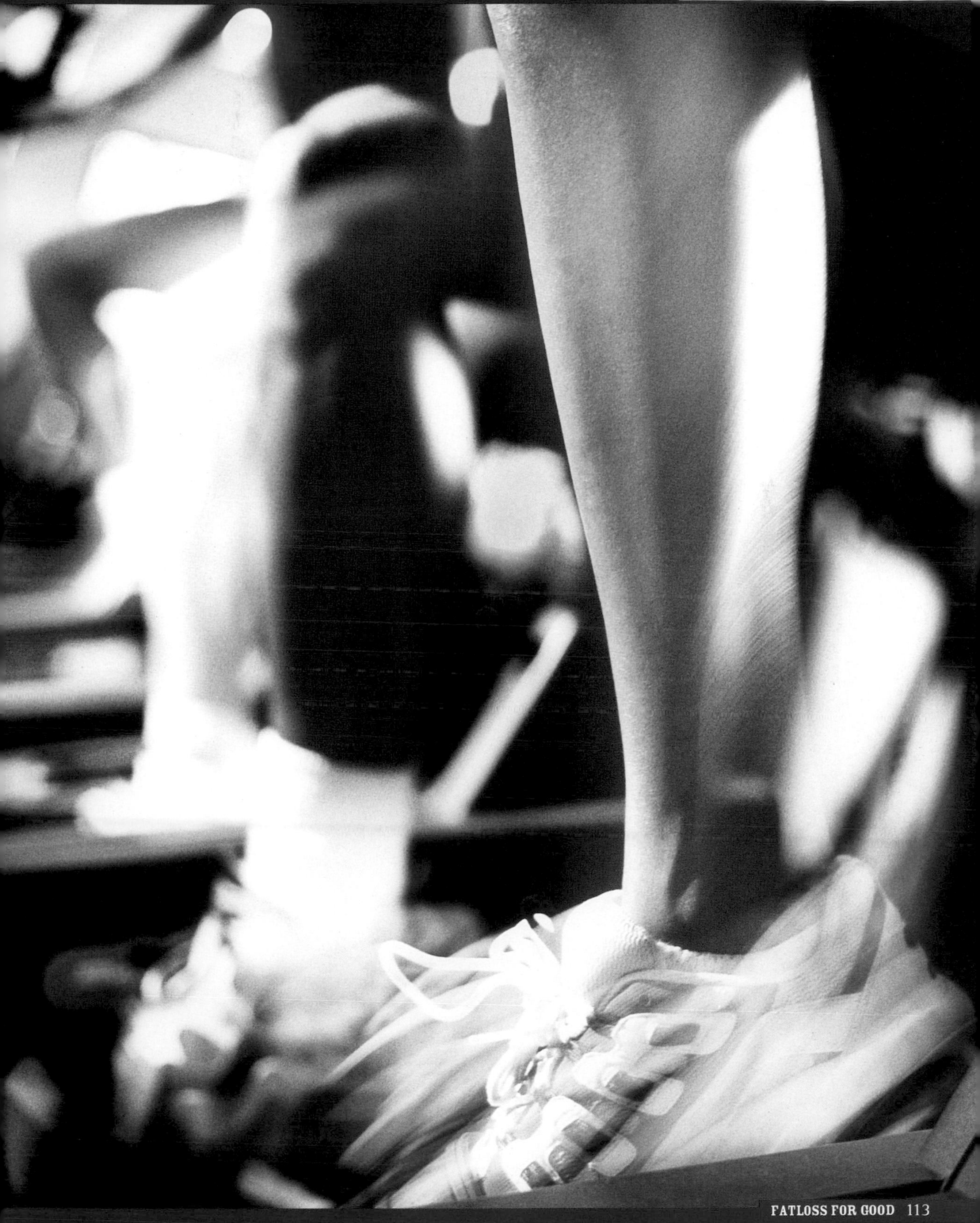

'The best way is to stress out your inner gladiator is to diet.

Kill or be killed

A gladiator knows all too well that good health is a life and death struggle. Here are the 12 most common preventable causes of death – tick them off your health list:

1. Smoking
2. High blood pressure
3. Obesity
4. Alcohol abuse
5. Low omega-3 fatty acids
6. High saturated fat intake
7. Low polyunsaturated fat intake
8. Salt punching not pinching
9. Low intake of fruits and vegies
10. Physical inactivity
11. High fasting blood glucose
12. High LDL cholesterol

> **TIFFINY'S EPIPHANY**
>
> Scales are only good for the kitchen. Ditch the body scales for food scales to measure your portions – and buy a calorie counter.

The diet corset

So many women have worn the corset of fad dieting for a lifetime – sucking the energy, colour and comfort from their lives. Dieting is a form of oppression that keeps us striving for a goal weight to distract us from the real issues plaguing our hearts – our lack of happiness, self-esteem and increased stress. Many of us couldn't imagine life without wearing this corset – it's been years – we only know life on a diet or off a diet. If we're not dieting, then what?

Dieting is defeatist. It's about depriving rather than giving – this isn't a warrior mindset!

Defeatist attitude: I can't eat that!

Warrior attitude: There is nothing I deny myself. I can eat anything I want, but I honour my body with healthy choices. I choose when to eat it and I will eat it only when I feel like it.

I want to liberate you from the diet corset strangling your mind. It's not just about gaining a healthy body by changing your eating habits rather than fad dieting; it's about establishing a healthy relationship with food – and with yourself.

Diets suck

When you go on a diet, your body changes its chemistry to make it easier to store fat in the future. As soon as your body senses a severe plummet in calories, your body holds back on pumping out thyroid hormone, resulting in a snail-paced metabolism.

Fad diets in particular can cause irreversible damage: they throw your hormones out of whack, eat away muscle mass and alter your biochemistry and brain chemistry to starve fat and crave sugar.

Diets suck even more when the starvation response kicks in and your body stops burning calories in order to conserve energy. Instinctively, your body will trigger your appetite hormones to try to force you to eat. Cravings will ensue, and good luck trying to defend yourself against them!

Scale new heights of confidence

Scales aren't a true indicator of fat loss – so ditch 'em! Scales measure weight – water, lean muscle mass and fat. Muscle is heavier than fat, so if you've built up your biceps, you'll weigh more on the scales. And if you're bloated, you'll weigh more from water retention.

Scales can't tell you what type of weight you've gained – those water gains at that time of the month, for example – or indeed what type of loss. You don't need to know your weight; what you *do* need to know is your measurements and fat loss percentage.

DIETS ARE DANGEROUS

In Australia, 68 per cent of 15-year-old girls are on a diet. Of these, 8 per cent are severely dieting. Adolescent girls who diet only moderately are five times more likely to develop an eating disorder than those who don't.

If you start dieting before the age of 15, you are more likely to experience depression, binge eating, purging and physical symptoms such as tiredness, low iron levels and menstrual irregularities. High-frequency and early onset of dieting are associated with poorer physical and mental health, eating disorders, extreme body dissatisfaction and more frequent general health problems. Women who diet frequently (that is, they've been on a diet more than five times) are 75 per cent more likely to experience depression.

The easiest way to see your weight loss progress is to use a favourite pair of jeans as your *perfect fit*. If you still fit 'em – you're all good. If they ever get tight – clean up your act foodwise and get exercising. You won't know success unless you measure your results, so have a friendly catch-up with a tape measure once a month to measure your thighs, hips, waist and bust.

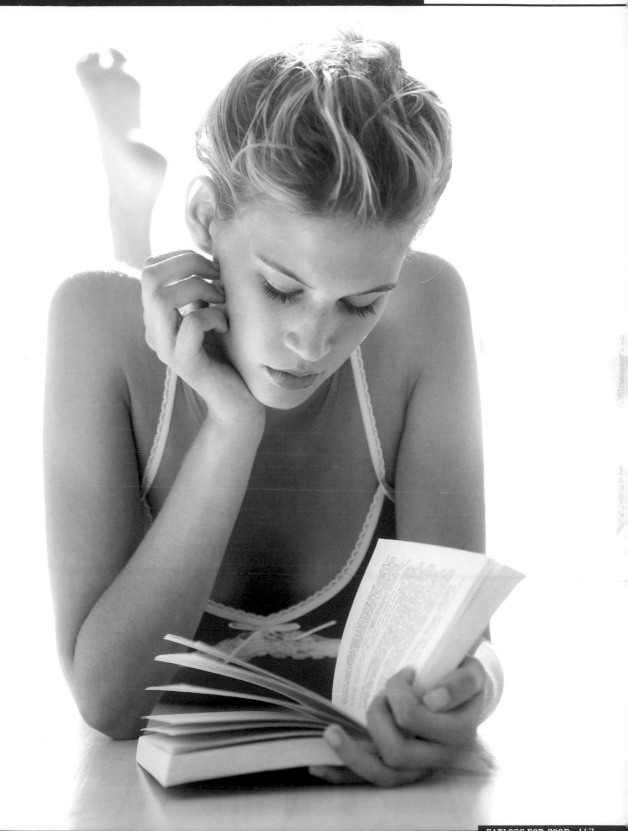

Apaches never miss their aim. Their **aim is true** because they know that success lies in the **preparation** for battle. Fail to prepare, and you prepare to fail.

Prepare to win the **battle**

i am apache warrior

protection

The overfeeding instinct

The apache warriors were instinctive eaters. When the hunt was on for food, the apaches would sometimes travel for an entire day without eating. And when they did eat, they had no way of knowing where their next meal would come from. This was instinctive eating.

Nowadays we have no need to overeat, yet when we see food our instinct is to store up goodies for the winter. Our bodies are instinctively designed to want to overeat, then physiologically designed to store that food as energy: fat.

The instinct to stop overeating

Our instinct may be to overeat, but we can also instinctively stop eating. Here's the cue: once you reach the point where you feel more thirsty than hungry, that's when you need to **start drinking and stop eating**.

When your body is dehydrated, your metabolism slows down, the fat-burning process stalls, toxins are no longer eliminated and nutrients aren't absorbed. And here's where our inner Apache Warrior needs to help, because it can be hard to recognise when we're thirsty. Instead of drinking, we respond by overeating, and that's where the danger lies.

Why do we put on weight?

We put on weight because we don't get enough exercise, right? Wrong. You won't lose weight by exercise alone. Exercise can help keep muscles toned, but losing fat is all about the food you eat. It's about good nutrition — you will always lose more weight by controlling what goes into your mouth than by exercising.

In a gym class, you can expect to burn up to 500 calories (2088 kJ), if you're working hard. Eat an apricot scroll with your morning coffee, and you're back to zero. No weight loss. Zilch. If you ran a marathon, you'd only burn 2600 calories (10,855 kJ) — that's the equivalent of a couple of double whopper burgers.

Are you prepared to bust a gut exercising to compensate for eating a large fast-food meal? We burn around 100 calories (418 kJ) an hour just hanging out and doing nothing. If it came down to choosing between exercise and food control as a form of weight management, I'd choose food every time, because it's faster and more effective.

EXERCISE DOESN'T EQUAL WEIGHT LOSS – GO FIGURE!

Good nutrition helps you to lose weight. Exercise helps to shape your body.

I once coached two overweight families and tried two different methods. One family ate a different diet for three weeks. The second family exercised intensely twice a day but stuck to their original diet.

Guess who had the best results? The family who changed what they ate and didn't exercise. The family who exercised actually put on weight, because they were more hungry.

The best way to lose weight is with food because it heats up your metabolism through digestion. It's impossible to catch up with exercise if you eat the wrong stuff.

apache warrior newsflash

If you up the ante to losing 200 calories (835 kJ) a day by eating less or moving more, you could lose up to 9.5 kg in one year!

100 calories (418 kJ)

The difference between weight loss and weight gain can be as little as 100 calories (418 kJ) a day.

My *Biggest Loser* contestants always tell me that their weight just 'crept' up on them. Many Australians experience this 'weight creep' – those nagging kilos that sneak on at an average of about 2 kilos per year. That's 20 kilos in 10 years!

The weight-maintenance remedy could be as simple as cutting out 100 calories (418 kJ) a day from your daily intake or adding 100 calories (418 kJ) a day to your daily exercise routine – or a combination of both if you're a Health Apache!

Keep it real

It's hard *not* to lose weight on Camp Biggest Loser – hours of exercise, 24-hour medical supervision, trainers at your beck-and-call, and a controlled environment with zero junk food available. Contestants on the show will lose anything between 4 and 10 kilos a week! This is not a realistic target for you. You should aim to lose half a kilo to 1 kilo a week – this is a healthy and achievable weightloss goal.

To achieve this, you need to save 500 calories (2088 kJ) a day. This could be two lattes a day or your morning muffin – sorry, cake!

'You are not on *The Biggest Loser.* Your weightloss goals need to be realistic.'

Go for good carbs

Your body and brain run on carbohydrates. Cut them out, and you'll feel moody, depleted, flat and unmotivated. So swear off the bad processed carbs and swear by the good stuff: oats, sweet potatoes, rye, sourdough, wholemeal breads and wholewheat pasta.

apache warrior newsflash

BURN CALORIES

Your metabolism converts food to energy. Just how fast or how slow depends on your lifestyle and how much lean body mass you carry. Remember that muscle burns up to 400 calories (1670 kJ) per kilo, so if you move more than you chew, your metabolism will burn baby burn!

It's all in the hormones

Instead of focusing on workouts at the gym, I believe there are four culprits that makes us fat:

1. Stress fat
2. Phantom fat = fructose
3. Overeating
4. Not targeting your eating to your hormones

We've already discussed the top three culprits, so let's throw a tomahawk at the hormones.

First off: I'm here to tell you there's no such thing as a fast or slow metabolism – metabolisms are either hormonally balanced or imbalanced.

Hormonal imbalances can cause obesity, accelerated ageing, depression, diabetes, certain forms of cancer, high cholesterol, heart disease, gout and sleep disorders. All this frightening stuff can be axed by taking the right medicine: the right food. By eating a nutritious diet, you can harmonise your body's hormones and balance your mind.

Different hormones are in charge of different functions – metabolic function, body fat composition, energy level, immunity and anti-ageing.

Insulin – the fat hormone

Insulin's gig is to clean your blood of sugar and store energy in fat cells.

Apache warriors had to run around the desert eating one meal a day if they were lucky, but there's no reason for you to skip meals. To keep your body's insulin working for you, you need to eat every four hours.

Remember 3, 2, 1: three meals, two snacks and at least 1 litre of water a day.

Fat storage is tied to the cyclical 'feast or famine' mentality of our forebears. When you eat meals four hours apart, your blood doesn't have a chance to miss food. The mere act of eating and digesting accounts for 10 per cent of your body's metabolic rate – Fatloss Warriors can't afford to cheat themselves out of that calorie burn! Feed your body regularly and it doesn't hold onto food for energy – it burns it, happy in the knowledge that it will soon be fed again.

TIFFINY'S EPIPHANY

Harness your inner Apache Warrior and target your eating to kill these hormone-snatching criminals!

Eating regularly also keeps your hunger hormones behaving. Leptin and ghrelin are the culprits that provoke you into a food frenzy. They're so powerful that they can actually make food taste up to 20 per cent better. What naughty ninjas!

apache warrior
move

One of the best foods to eat to reverse age-related deficits in memory and learning are blueberries. They are high in flavonoids that provide antioxidant protection. Antioxidants are critical to healthy neurogenesis. Add these blue bubbles of brain power to smoothies, breakfast bowls, salads, freeze 'em an' suck 'em, and bake them into your healthy savory muffins.

CALORIE COUNT

1 gram of fat = 9 calories (38 kJ)
1 gram of carbohydrate & protein = 4 calories (17 kJ)
1 gram of alcohol = 7 calories (29 kJ)

Thyroid – the calorie-counting hormone

Thyroid hormones perform the whole apache artillery of body functions – they control the amount of oxygen each cell uses, your heart rate, body temperature, fertility, digestion, mood and, most importantly, the rate at which your body burns calories.

Thyroid imbalances are common, and the symptoms – changes in energy, mood and weight – are similar to many other conditions. Many people have a thyroid imbalance without knowing it.

Thyroid thugs

Some of the following foods are super good for you, so only avoid 'em if you're sure you have a thyroid problem.

- Diets – swear off diets forever!
- Caffeine – coffee, tea, chocolate, soft drinks, energy drinks
- Cruciferous vegetables – brussels sprouts, cauliflower, mustard, turnips, bok choy, horseradish
- Zapping carbs – refined grains, white breads, pasta, sugar, potatoes, baked goods, corn
- Pine nuts, bamboo shoots, strawberries, radishes, peaches
- Soy – tempeh, tofu, fake meat products

Testosterone – the toning hormone

TIFFINY'S EPIPHANY

Do you eat after 9 pm? If so, cork it after 8 pm.

Think of testosterone and we think of bodybuilders, bar bawls and back hair, but testosterone doesn't only benefit dudes. These hormones can give women more energy, motivate us to hit the gym, and help us build more calorie-burning muscle. But don't worry, ladies – boosting your testosterone won't make you bulky. Rather, it'll help tone and shape your body: no more back cleavage, kankles, overhanging bra fat or bingo wings – thanks, testosterone!

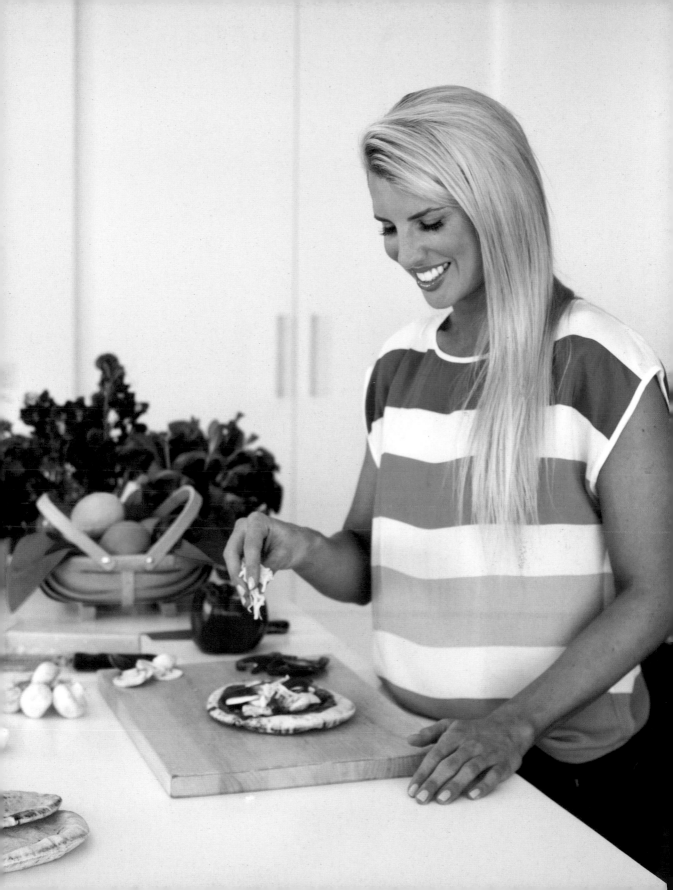

Toning hormones are anabolic hormones – that is, they're forces of good in the metabolic war, building rather than destroying. Testosterone increases lean muscle mass and strength, boosts libido and improves energy.

Testosterone tragics

- Low-fat diets – a low-fat diet can block the normal rise in testosterone after lifting weights, so make sure your post-exercise snack has a decent amount of good fats and protein
- Low-protein diets – try to make your meal 30–40% protein
- Alcohol – reduces testosterone, especially in men
- Licorice – I hate this because licorice is my favourite treat, but it blocks the enzymes responsible for creating testosterone. The occasional piece of black rope won't hurt but don't make it a comfort food.
- Stress
- Vitamin deficiencies

Estrogen – the mood hormone

Estrogen helps stabilise mood and keep your energy levels high. It also lowers your insulin and blood pressure levels, raises HDL ('good') cholesterol and lowers LDL ('bad') cholesterol.

Weight issues creep up as women approach menopause because their production of estrogen decreases, prompting another type of estrogen – estrone – to play a larger role. Estrone causes the body to hang onto fat, especially in the belly.

Estrogen equations

- Increase your dietary fibre – the more fibre, the better your natural estrogen system works
- Eat your broccoli and cabbage – cruciferous vegies have antioxidants that help to reduce the risk of breast and cervical cancers
- Power with pomegranate – it's believed to help prevent prostate cancer cells, so get ya pom juice, boys!

Cortisol – the stress hormone

Our bodies are designed for stress. When we were apache warriors being hunted by wild animals, our stress hormones relaxed our stomach muscles and decreased the blood flow to our intestines, allowing us to outrun the bear instead of digesting our food. Once the stress had passed, cortisol then told our bodies to stop producing the stress hormones and to resume digestion.

apache warrior move
STRESSSED OUT
Keep yourself in high-stress mode, and you set yourself up for heart disease, diabetes, stroke and other potentially fatal conditions.

Problem is, these days we wrestle with all kinds of beasts – mortgages, hellish jobs, family problems, overbooked schedules. We can't always outrun them, and that's what keeps us wired all the time. If the stressor never goes away, cortisol hangs around and continues to stimulate our appetites. You know what I'm talking about – you feel stressed, so you crave high-fat, high-carb foods. And once you eat, your body floods your brain with happy chemicals that can set up an addictive relationship with food.

When cortisol levels remain high, the body actually resists weight loss. Cortisol also turns young fat cells into mature fat cells that hang on for dear life. To make matters worse, cortisol tends to create fat where you least want it – around your tummy.

EATING IN THE DARK

Do you only eat lunchfast? That is, skip breakfast and not eat until lunchtime? When you're asleep, lack of food makes your metabolism slow down. Breakfast breaks the fast of sleeping and kickstarts your metabolism for the day.

If you skip meals throughout the day, you'll end up consuming most of your calories at night. Eating in the dark is dangerous because you're generally less active in the evening and so you tend to store more calories. Close the kitchen after dinner to avoid constant snacking, and try to make your last meal for the day high in protein and sans sugar to keep your insulin levels down.

Cortisol criminals

- Alcohol – activates the adrenal glands, forcing them to spit out more cortisol
- Caffeine – elevates cortisol secretion, so moderation is key: up to 200 mg of caffeine a day, total
- Gluten – try gluten-free products or just try to reduce the amount of wheat products you consume, as gluten intolerance leads to increased cortisol levels
- Licorice – it inhibits an enzyme that deactivates cortisol in the kidneys
- Salt – since 80% of our sodium comes from eating processed foods, switch to eating naked to help you stay in the safe range: 6 grams of sodium a day
- Stress
- Depression
- Skipping breakfast
- Fad diets

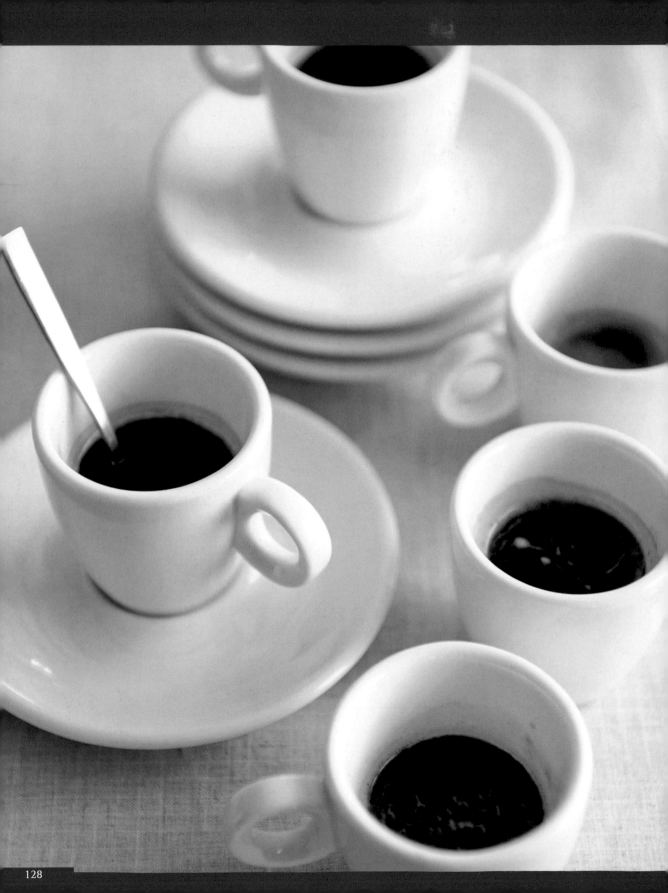

Leptin – the full hormone

Leptin is a kind of fat-cell hormone that's released when you've eaten a meal. Its job is to travel to your brain and tell it, 'I'm full!' Leptin also switches on other appetite-suppressing signals, so your body gets the message to stop being hungry and start burning more calories – a great message.

When it's working right, leptin helps the body tap into longer-term fat stores – it helps burn off those saddle bags and muffin tops that have been there for years. But when leptin signalling gets screwy, your brain never receives the 'I'm stuffed!' signal and you overeat.

Leptin leeches

- Eating all your calories in one sitting – a massive dinner will delay the release of leptin until two hours after you've finished eating. Remember to spread your meals out over the day, separated by four-hour intervals.
- High-fat junk food – rubbish fast food will block leptin and increase your cravings and appetite. It's called trash for a reason!
- Fructose – unlike other sugars, fructose doesn't stimulate insulin, and it's invisible. If leptin doesn't know the fructose is in your system, it can't get to work. Soft drinks and lollies are the worst, but also be mindful to keep your fruit down to a maximum of three pieces a day.
- Alcohol – your body scrapes up leptin and chucks it in the kidneys with the turps!
- Caffeine – that caffè latte blocks leptin, and you don't want to roadblock the hormone that regulates your appetite and stops you from eating, do you?

apache warrior newsflash
FAT CELLS

Fat cells are more than blobs of yuck waiting to get bigger or smaller. The fat in your body is an enormous endocrine gland, actively reacting to your body's hormones.

What is gluten?

Gluten is a protein that's found in grains like wheat, barley and rye. Most of us are in love with gluten without knowing it. After all, it goes into making our favourite things like bread and thick gloopy sauces. You can be allergic to gluten, so if you're having gut issues, see a specialist.

Ghrelin – the hunger hormone

Ghrelin is the shoe to your leptin laces. Just as leptin tells your brain to turn off hunger, ghrelin tells your brain that you're famished. Ghrelin is the reason you always feel hungry at particular moments in the day – your body clock triggers its release according to a finely tuned schedule. Ghrelin is also released whenever your stomach is empty, and levels will stay elevated until you've given your body enough nutrients to satisfy its needs. Satiety signals can take some time to kick in, that's why eating slowly can help you eat less.

Ghrelin gangsters

- Low-calorie foods – they'll only make you hungrier! Don't be tempted to lose weight quickly. Ditch those replacement drinks, bars and diets, and your hunger hormone won't be so savage.
- Fructose – ghrelin rises after you ingest fructose because it doesn't think you've eaten anything. Fruit makes you feel hungrier!
- Low-protein foods – fats don't suppress ghrelin nearly as well as carbs or protein, which may be another reason why high-fat diets lead to weight gain. Bad fats such as deep-fried foods, ice-cream and junk food – you know what foods I'm talking about – will make you a Naughty Ninja! Get ya Apache Warrior on instead!
- Binge foods – as soon as you smell your favourite junk foods, ghrelin is released along with your stomach juices in preparation for an influx of sugar. Any high-sugar, high-calorie food that tempts you will cause you to overeat. Those cakes, lollies, freshly baked cookies and Boston buns that seem to scream at you from across the street or down the supermarket aisles – these are trigger foods, and if you struggle with binge eating, you have to learn to go cold turkey. Quit straight up!
- Alcohol – you know the drill by now: drinking beer, wine and spirits will make you a munching monster.
- Eating in the dark – snacking at night raises ghrelin levels and will keep you awake. You need lower ghrelin levels to sleep, so put your food nightcap on at 8 pm.

The Dynamite Dozen

Change your brain and transform your body with my 12 Apache Warrior targets.

1. **What you see in the mirror is your brain** – you are everything you think, so remember the importance of monitoring your brain hygiene.
2. **If you can't get motivated to exercise, stick to healthy eating.** If you're low on energy and drive, then don't start at the gym – exercise your mental health in your Mind Gym.
3. **R.E.S.P.E.C.T. your brain**, and eat right to stay bright. Your brain uses 25 per cent of the calories you consume, 25 per cent of the total blood flow in your body and 20 per cent of the oxygen you breathe. Forget crash diets, punishing exercise, dangerous supplements – what's important is the health of your brain. Get into brain foods, like almonds, avocados, cranberries, grapefruit, kiwi fruit, lentils, pomegranates, tofu and walnuts.
4. **Drugs and alcohol** – give them the flick 'cos they cause your appetite to fluctuate drastically, causing weight gain or loss. They also sap your motivation and energy, and can lead to long-term brain damage.

5. **Obesity** – fat stores toxic materials in the brain and doubles the risk of Alzheimer's disease. A double no-no.

6. **Malnutrition** – your body renews the cells in your body every few months. These new cells draw on all the foods you consume, so you really are what you eat. A trashy diet will buy you a trashy brain.

7. **Chronic stress** – constant stress tells your body to release higher levels of the stress hormone, cortisol, leading to a voracious appetite, demonic cravings and chronic pain.

8. **Sleep deprivation** – anything less than six hours a night lowers overall brain function and causes your brain to secrete hormones that amp up your appetite and cravings for white food and sugary snacks. People who sleep less, eat more.

9. **Smoking** – nicotine constricts the blood flow to the brain and the organs in your body, including your skin – that's why smokers wrinkle up. Smokers' brains look that way too.

10. **Dehydration** – your body consists of 70 per cent water and your brain is 80 per cent water. If you don't drink, your brain shrinks.

11. **Lack of exercise** – when you don't exercise, the blood flow to your brain is decreased.

12. **Negative thinking** – focusing on negative thoughts lowers brain activity, causes your heart to beat faster and increases blood pressure. Negative thoughts lead to negative physical effects.

BINGE BLOAT

Don't freak out if you have a binge. Sometimes it just happens – a big night, stress, or maybe you just wanted to eat! If you weigh yourself the next day, don't go ballistic if you've put on an extra few kilos. It's natural for a female to gain up to 3 kilos after an increased carbohydrate intake because for every gram of carbohydrate you consume, the body will store 3 grams of water. As long as you get back to healthy eating and exercise the next day, those extra kilos will disappear over 48 hours.

Stop stress at work

Let's face it, the workplace can be a stressful environment. Here are some ideas to release the stress lever and ward off those unfriendly allies of stress: binge eating, depression, dehydration and soaring cortisol levels.

- **Learn to say NO!** When something extra is asked of you at work, weigh up what it will cost you financially, emotionally, physically and intellectually. If the stress outweighs the benefits, bow out.

BRAIN BEAUTIFIERS

- Hydration
- Mental health
- Healthy diet
- Balanced hormones
- Multivitamins
- Fish oil
- Deep breathing

- Relaxation
- Communication
- Meditation
- Sleep
- Learning
- Exercise
- Gratitude

- **Don't eat it up but talk it out** – remember that you're not alone. Talking to family or friends will help you to vent. Plus, they may be able to come up with a solution to the problem that is causing you so much stress at work.
- **Know your triggers.** Do you get nervous when you drink too much coffee, or when you have to speak to a certain group of people? Make a very specific list of your stress trigger points and hot spots. Figure out how you can change these things so they no longer pose a problem for you.
- **Create a de-stress toolbox for your desk:** choose a favourite CD, picture, quote or poem. Include healthy snacks, aromatherapy oils, vitamins, a water bottle, soothing pawpaw cream, a selection of calming herbal teas and a hand moisturiser.
- **Keep plants in the office** – they increase oxygen so you can think more clearly.
- **Exercise plays a key role** in reducing and preventing the effects of stress, by helping to relax muscle tension and improve sleep. When stress is peaking, get up and move. Take a walk around the parking lot or do some stretches at your desk. Away from work, yoga, tai chi and martial arts are excellent stress-busters. You gotta move to improve!
- **Try my 5 Year Test.** Whenever I am *really* stressed out about something, I gain a sense of perspective by asking myself: will this matter in five years' time? Or even five months from now? If it won't matter then, it's not worth stressing out over now.
- **Make an appointment with fun!** Schedule yourself some free time and give yourself something to look forward to.
- **Shallow breathing is a common response to stress,** depriving the body of adequate oxygen and preventing you from thinking clearly and functioning properly. The next time you feel stressed, take five or six long, deep breaths – in through your nose and out through your mouth. Your body will respond with reduced muscle tension, lower blood pressure and slower heart rate.

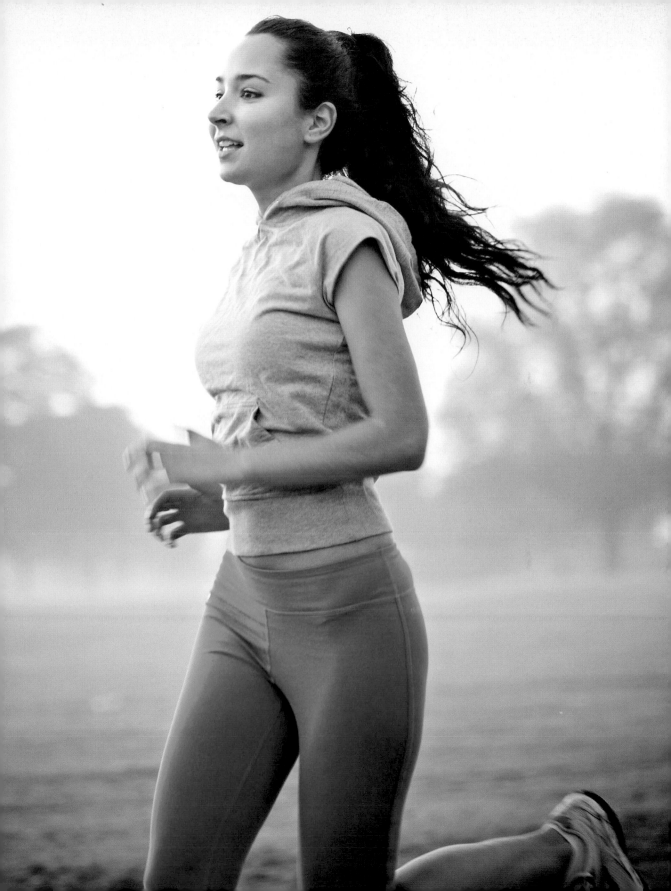

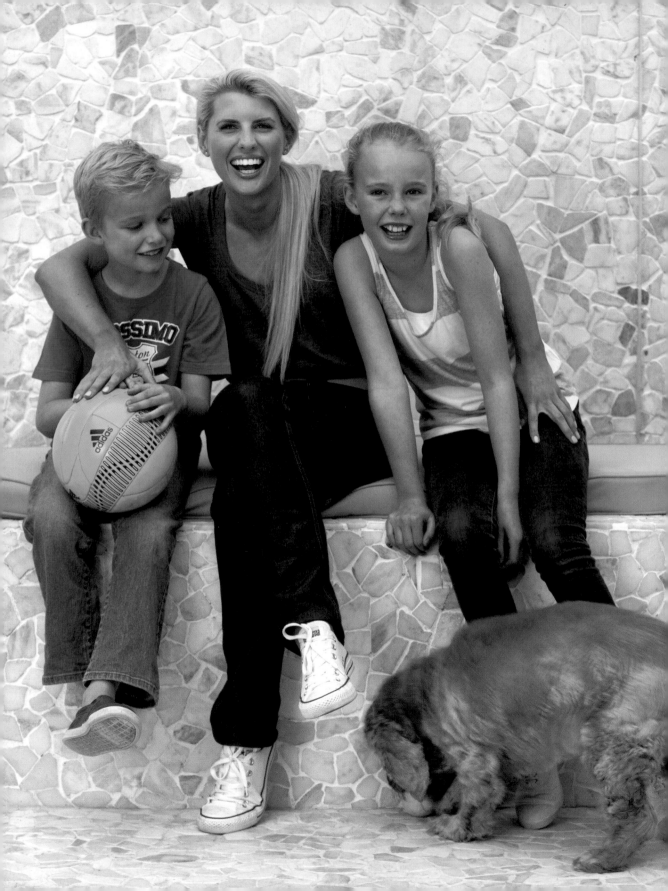

- **Find a hobby.** When your job has built up to be too much for you to handle, relax and release the tension by finding something you enjoy doing. A hobby will allow you to spend some quiet time with yourself in calm surroundings.
- **We've always heard that laughter is the best medicine**, now we have proof. Laughter reduces stress by releasing endorphins that lower your blood pressure, stimulate your brain, release tight muscles, change your emotional landscape and increase your oxygen intake.
- **Chemicals like caffeine, nicotine, alcohol and sugar spike energy short term, but can make things worse in the long run.** Try to limit their use during the day and especially before you go to bed.

Axe sugar from your kids' diet

Children learn all about food from who else but you. I reckon lesson Number One is teaching our kids the difference between regular food and party food.

When I lived with my obese *Biggest Loser* family, one of the biggest shocks for me was discovering that they ate party food *every single day*. Family blocks of chocolate, party pies, lollies, family packs of Doritos, soft drinks, popcorn – this family ate treats like food! A regular night in front of the TV doesn't classify as a party. So don't keep junk in the house: don't buy junk and don't eat junk at home. Party foods should only be for special occasions.

Apache Warrior tips for little angels

- Read the labels on your kids' foods – even baby foods can have added sugar.
- Rather than having cold, sweetened cereals for breakfast, serve hot, unsweetened breakfast cereals such as plain oatmeal, and add raisins or fresh fruit.
- Freeze grapes, blueberries, banana, peaches and strawberries as sweet healthy snacks.
- Serve a small serving of dessert with the main meal instead of later in the evening, when your kids are more likely to overeat mindlessly in front of the TV.
- Make your own baked goods at home and cut the amount of sugar called for in the recipe by half.
- Ban chocolate spreads and replace them with smashed avocado on bread.
- Rubbish the fruit roll-ups and replace them with real fruit. Or purée some fruit, then bake it and rip it into fruit leather strips.
- Chuck processed cheese sticks and replace them with cubes of real cheese sliced off the block.
- Boycott 'kids' yoghurts that could classify as confectionery and freeze your own full-fat natural Jalna yoghurts. Plain yoghurt and fruit contains natural, not added sugars.
- Choose water or plain milk over soft drinks.

Tots' tastebud taekwondo

Kids' foods are loaded with heaps of added sugar and sodium, and their colour scheme is beige (think fries, nuggets, white bread, low-fibre cereals) – but the good news is it's never too late to retrain your kids' sweet, salty and bland tastebuds. Tastebuds regenerate every three to ten days, so your kids can grow a healthier set!

Kids need five or six tries at tasting something new before they'll decide if they like it, so hang in there! The most important part of Tastebud Taekwondo is diligence. To entice your little ninjas to try new foods, encourage them to help out in your dish dojang – the kitchen.

- Try out different recipes and food combinations – if it smells great and your kids help you to cook it, then they will be more tempted to eat their masterpiece. Your kids can wash and scrub the vegetables, or peel and toss a salad together.
- Try introducing one new vegetable a week and make new tastes fun by giving the vegie a super power. Carrots to give you X-ray vision. Spinach to make you strong. Sweet potato mash to make you fast. Asparagus to make you smart.
- If your kids aren't yet ready for super powers, try the rule of bites – one bite for every year. By the time your kids are getting towards seven and eight, they'll no longer be thinking in bites, they'll just be eating their vegetables!
- Mash doesn't have to be white – you can mash green peas, sweet potato, cauliflower or corn.
- Cut fruit into shapes: stars, moons, rainbows. They always taste better!

The Gym of Life

Exercise is a new invention. Back when there were neither cars nor computers and only caves, mountains and uncharted terrain, we had to move in order to survive. Even when there weren't any immediate threats, there was the need to gather food and provide shelter. A heap of activity was built into the normal course of the day – everyone was an athlete!

We invented exercise out of necessity. If we didn't spend most of our time being sedentary, then we wouldn't put on weight and need to exercise to burn it off. The secret is to keep moving throughout the day, and use energy efficiently. In other words, join the Gym of Life.

There are three types of movement:

Exercise – intentional exertion to maintain physical fitness.
Gym of life – movement that's built into the day, including walking, biking to work, taking the stairs, housework, gardening.
Mindful movement – an activity that requires greater awareness of the body, such as yoga or tai chi, or that involves learning skilled movements, such as dancing or martial arts.

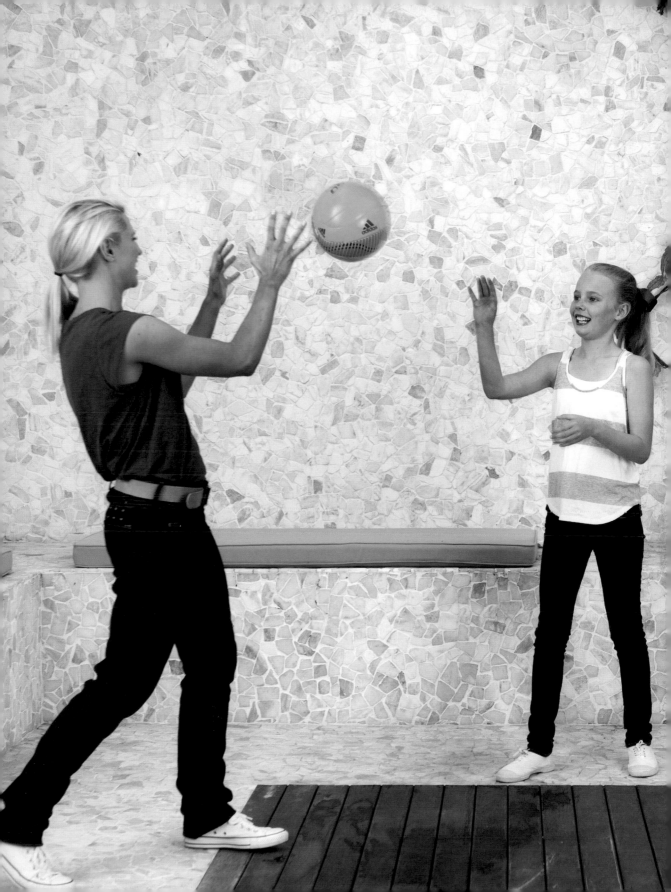

apache warrior
newsflash
GYM OF LIFE TIPS
Walk quickly, everywhere
Ditch the car!
Use the stairs
Walk several times around a
shopping centre
Vacuuming can work up a
sweat!

Moving your body lengthens your life expectancy and is one of the most powerful antidepressants there is. I find that martial arts teaches me to listen and connect with my body, so I can understand when I am feeling hungry, unhappy, hurt or low on energy. When you listen to your body, you then learn how to heal your body. Perhaps you don't need food but a friend to talk it out. Perhaps you don't need sleep but mentalaxation.

When it comes to stress, exercise does it all. It protects cells from oxidation, helps stabilise blood sugar, decreases inflammation, treats depression and promotes new brain cell survival, growth and learning. It even increases insulin receptors, helps normalise cortisol levels and boosts brain growth. Exercise is as much for the mind as it is for the body!

APACHE WARRIOR GYM OF LIFE

It's recommended that adults put in a minimum of 2 hours of intense aerobic activity per week. But if you only exercise a couple of hours a week, that leaves over 100 hours in the week when you're not exercising. You can see the problem …

We evolved to be moving most of the day – not exercising – but instead, we just sit. That's where the Gym of Life comes in. It's the extra movement we squeeze in without really realising it: pacing, using your hands to speak, fidgeting, taking the stairs, jumping over obstacles in our path, ducking branches.

It's an absolute fact that movement burns calories, and that people who are more mobile are less likely to be obese.

My advice is to exercise for at least 40 minutes every day: push your heart rate and sweat. In addition, activate your Gym of Life membership all day long. And be creative with your membership!

Gym of life for teens

If you want to exercise with your teens or twenty-somethings, mix walking or jogging with circuit training by stopping at park benches along the way to do sets of push-ups, dips, sit-ups and squats. Mother–daughter walks are important because 30 minutes a day decreases the risk of breast cancer by 30 per cent.

Setting shared weight-loss and fitness goals – like completing a 5-kilometre swim or a half-marathon – can also get you moving with your tribe.

Interval success

The biggest movement myth out there is that to burn the most fat you have to suffer through long, arduous, boring sweaty slots of cardio. Wrong! You can triple your fat loss and shed kilos in killer time by incorporating intervals.

Interval training is how I stripped more than 10 kilos off my contestants in one week! As an example, studies showed that by mixing 8 seconds of fast pedalling

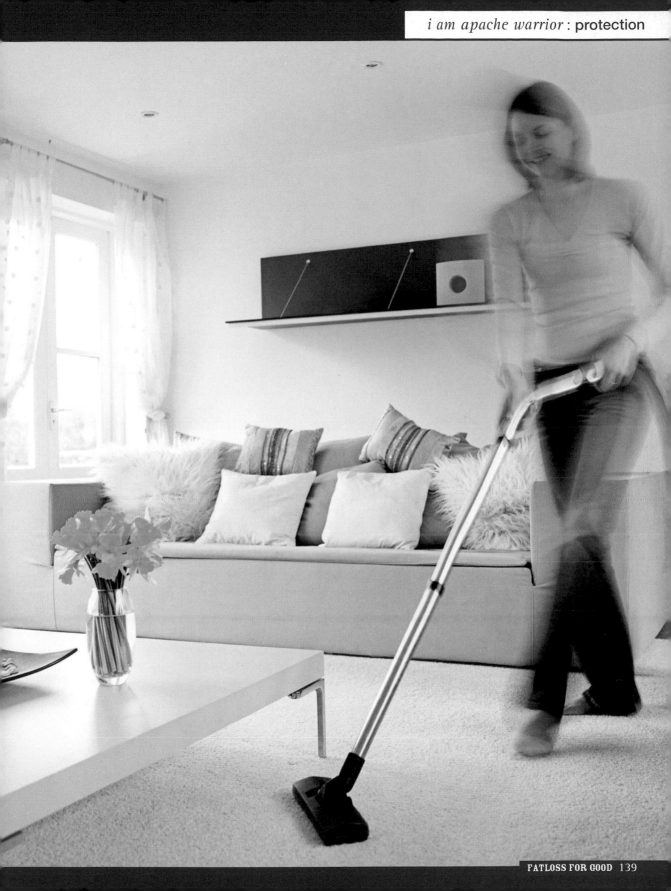

and 12 seconds of light pedalling over a 20-minute cycling workout, participants lost three times as much fat as those who exercised at a moderate pace for a full 40 minutes.

A cardio workout isn't the best way to burn fat. Resistance training – such as using free weights, your own body weight, resistance bands or gym machines – is better than dieting or even the dieting and cardio mix. Research shows that people who diet without exercising lose 69 per cent of their fat; people who diet and do cardio lose 78 per cent of their fat; and those who diet, do cardio and resistance training using weights burn 97 per cent of their fat – now that's really unleashing your inner Apache Warrior!

Interval training tips

I do 20 minutes of interval training every day: either running outside, boxing, sprints in my dojang, free weights or using the machines at the gym. In fact, you can use anything to do intervals and get your inner Apache Warrior fighting fit: weights, cross trainer, spin bike, walking, swimming or treadmill.

Try these two killer programs – keep it to 20 minutes though!

TREADMILL: 20-MINUTE INTERVAL PROGRAM

2 minutes: Raise the incline to 10 and keep your speed at anything between 4 and 9 km an hour, depending on your fitness. Run for 2 minutes flat stick.
1 minute: Increase the speed to 2 to 4 km an hour faster and sprint for 1 minute.
Go apache warrior, go!
2 minutes: Jog at a comfortable pace – that's slow enough for you to conduct a conversation – for 1 minute.
Total = 5 minutes
Repeat 4 times

SPIN BIKE: 12-MINUTE INTERVAL PROGRAM

2 minutes: Pedal at a hard pace that gets your legs moving and engages your core.
Rest interval
12 seconds: Sprint to 80% of your maximum heart rate.
Rest for 8 seconds
Repeat for 6 minutes: 12 seconds going hard, 8-second rest interval
2 minutes: Sprint, pushing your heart rate as high as it will go.
Go apache warrior, go!
Total = 12 minutes

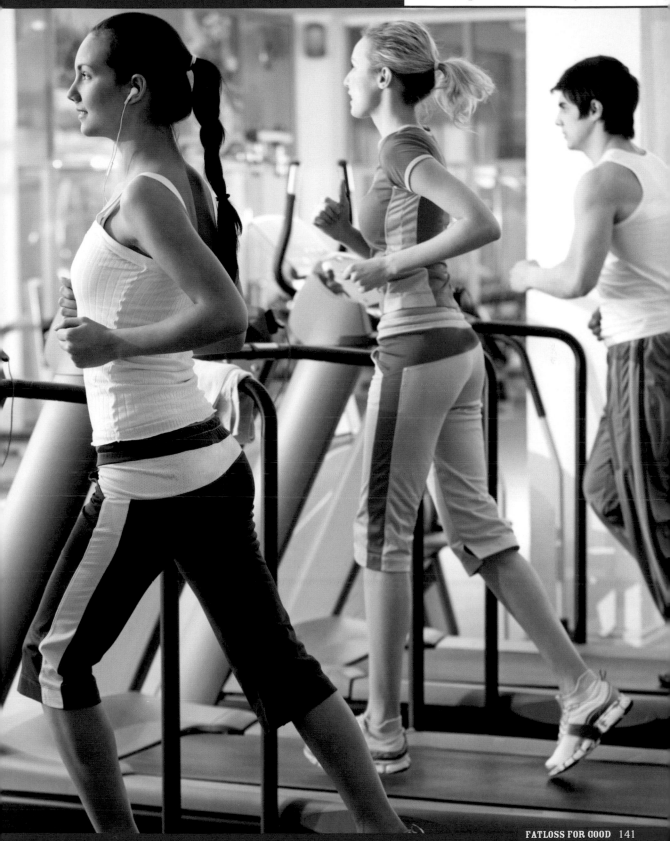

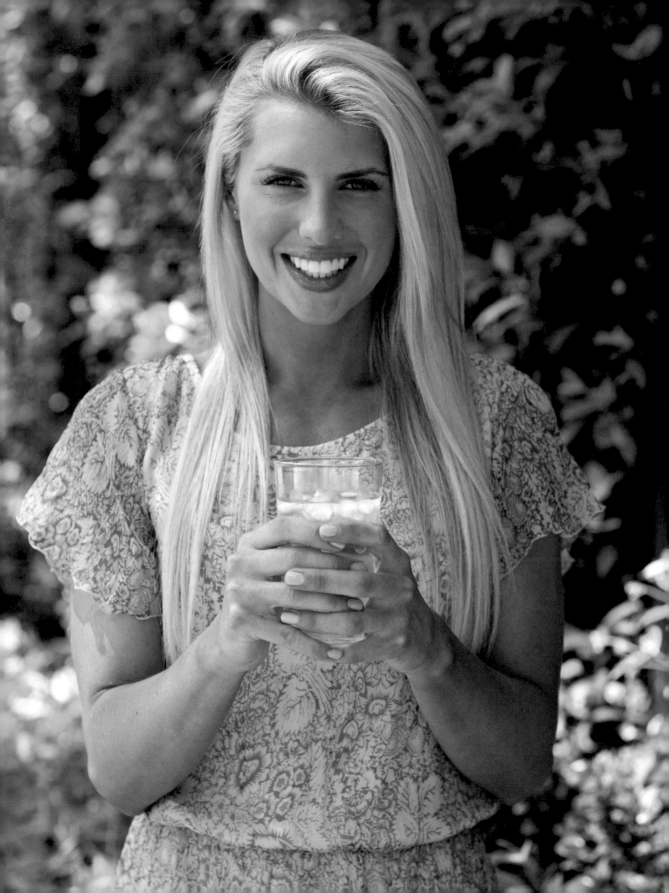

Resistance training program

Perform repetitions of the following exercises for 30 seconds, followed by a 10-second rest. Repeat each exercise four times.

- Pushups
- Dips
- Biceps curls with 1 litre carton of milk
- Lunges with phonebook

A last toast – drink up!

If you don't drink, you can't think. Coffee, tea, alcohol, energy drinks and soft drinks aren't substitutes for the natural water your body hungers and they won't quench your stressed-out body when it's dehydrated.

By the time you feel a symptom of dehydration, such as a headache, you have already lost up to a litre of water. And when you exercise, you need to drink at least an extra litre of water for every hour of exercise you do. 'Dry mouth' is the very last sign of dehydration, yet it's often the first thing we notice.

Most importantly, if you're dehydrated, you stall the fat burn process. So why do people put on weight? Simple: they don't know the difference between fluids and water.

I'm a non-drinker because I know that alcohol dehydrates you. It causes serious drought in your brain cells and puts your body under palpable stress. Alcohol is just not conducive to living a stress-free healthy life. Similarly, caffeine, soft drinks and teas are dehydrating agents because of their strong diuretic effect on the kidneys.

Before I even started to tackle the contestants' diets on *The Biggest Loser*, I began Water Therapy. My contestants needed to be able to distinguish hunger from thirst. By drinking water before eating food, they managed to separate the two sensations. My contestants then stopped overeating to satiate their thirst, and they began to drink water to combat their dehydration. Overeating was out, and hydration was in!

A final warrior **word ...**

Dear Ninjas,

I wrote this book because I believe our thoughts shape our world. We are not only what we eat, but also a creation of what we think. I know that in difficult times, when all seems lost and hopeless, the only thing that can rescue us is our mental strength.

We need to maintain our cognitive fitness just as diligently as we maintain our bodies. The brain is our lifeguard, our mentor and our companion.

Your health is worth fighting for, and you are now trained to combat not only unhealthy habits, but also junk thoughts. Using the stealth of the ninja, the control of the samurai, the awareness of the Shaolin monk, the strength of the gladiator and the protection of the apache, you can build yourself a healthier brain to map supportive habits and chart a brighter future.

TIFFINY'S EPIPHANY

Start with ninja stars – small change – before moving onto big changes – and soon those inch pebbles will become milestones.

My wish for you is that, with the support of your A-Team of Warriors, you can continue the Health Ninja journey for life.

GO NINJAS, GO NINJAS, GO!

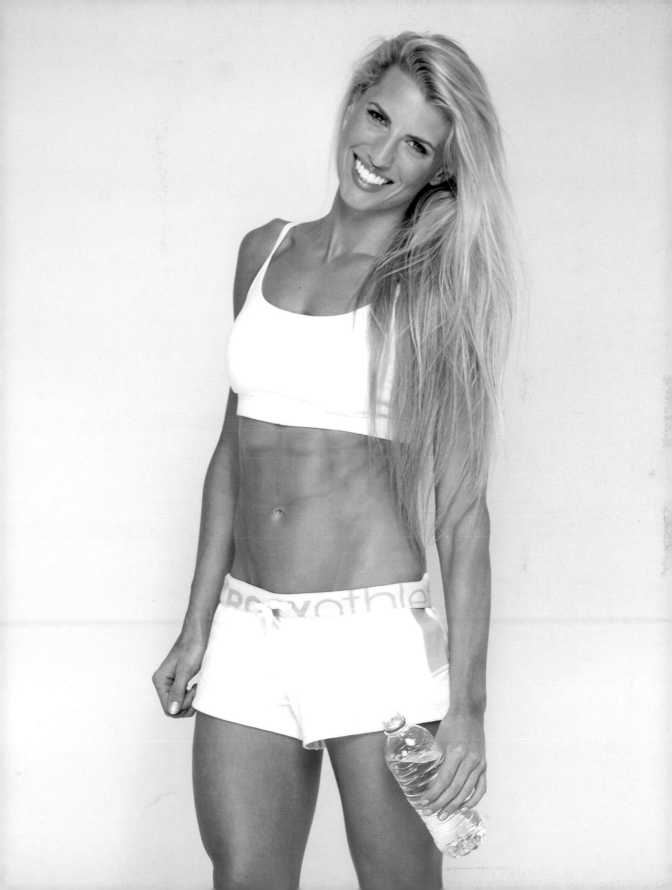

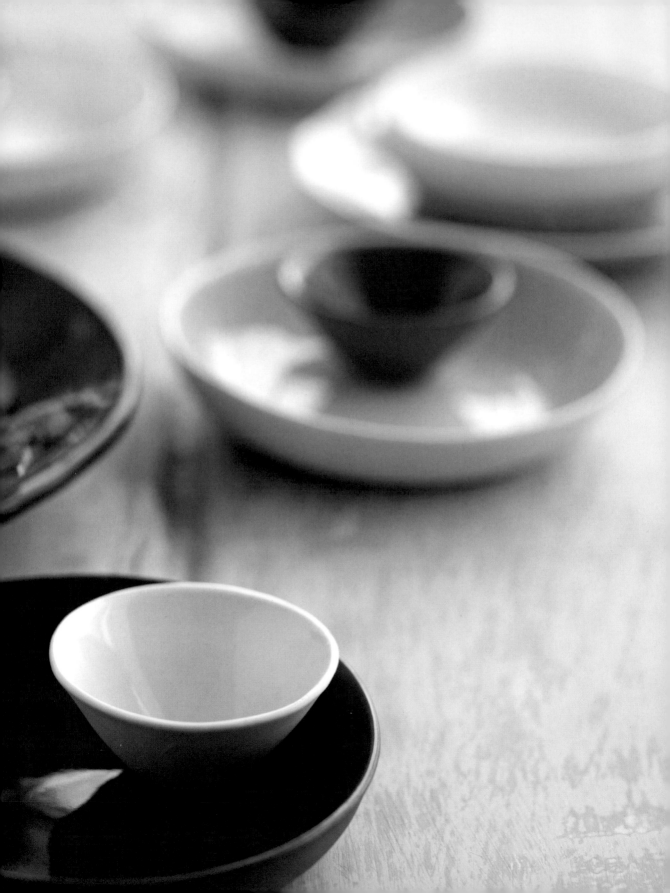

6

Feed your **soul**

recipes

Fast breakfast smoothie

SERVES 1

1 cup almond milk
¼ cup frozen mixed berries
1 tablespoon cocoa nibs

Combine all ingredients in a blender and mix until smooth.

Note: In case you haven't come across them before, cocoa nibs are pieces of hulled and roasted cacao beans. They're packed with magnesium, calcium, zinc, copper and potassium. You can find them at specialty food stores or good health food shops.

WAY TO START THE DAY!

Coconut quinoa porridge

SERVES 4

$1/2$ cup reduced-fat coconut milk

$1/2$ cup water

1 cup quinoa, rinsed

1 cup fresh raspberries

1 cup fresh blueberries

$1/2$ teaspoon ground cinnamon

4 teaspoons LSA
(LSA: ground linseed, sunflower, almond mix)

4 teaspoons agave nectar

Combine the coconut milk, water and quinoa in a medium saucepan and bring to the boil over a high heat. Reduce heat, cover and simmer for 10-12 minutes or until most of the liquid is absorbed. Turn off the heat and let stand, covered, for 5 minutes. Fluff the cooked quinoa with a fork and fold in the berries and cinnamon.

Top with LSA and a drizzle of agave nectar to serve.

GIVE IT A GO!

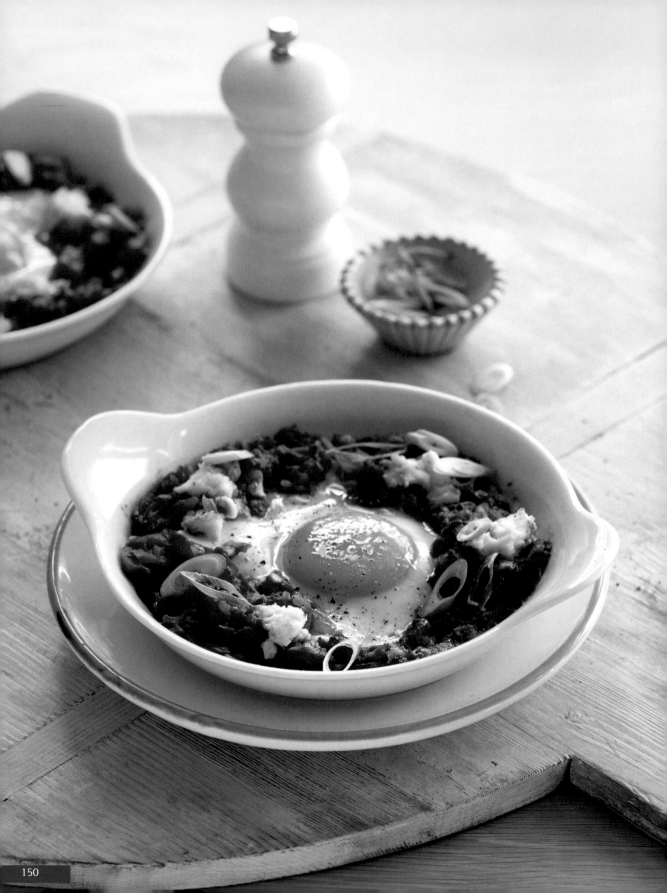

Spicy baked eggs

MAKES 4

1 tablespoon extra-virgin olive oil
1 onion, finely diced
½ red capsicum, sliced
1 garlic clove, minced
400 g can chopped tomatoes
½ teaspoon harissa paste
¼ cup water
4 eggs
4 tablespoons ricotta
½ cup spring onion, finely sliced

Preheat oven to 200ºC.

Sauté the onions in the oil over medium heat for 5 minutes,
then add the capsicum and garlic and cook for a further
2 minutes until the mixture is softened. Add the tomatoes, harissa
and water. Simmer for 10 minutes.

Divide the tomato mixture between four 250 ml ramekins.
Make a well in the centre of each dish and crack an egg into it.
Scatter the ricotta over the top and bake for
10-12 minutes, until the whites are just set. Garnish with
spring onion to serve.

GREAT BREAKFAST PROTEIN!

Spelt pancakes with ricotta, honey and toasted coconut

MAKES 8

4 tablespoons shredded coconut
1 cup spelt flour
2 teaspoons baking powder
pinch of cinnamon
pinch of salt
1 egg
1 cup buttermilk
1 tablespoon extra-virgin olive oil
2 tablespoons yoghurt
1 banana, sliced
drizzle of honey to serve

To toast the coconut, dry fry in a pan over medium heat until just starting to colour. Remove from heat and set aside.

Sift the flour, baking powder, cinnamon and salt into a large bowl. In a separate bowl, mix the egg and buttermilk. Pour the wet ingredients into the dry ingredients and gently fold until just combined.

Heat the oil in a frying pan over medium heat. Spoon in 2 tablespoons of the batter and cook until slightly golden. Turn over and cook through. Repeat with remaining batter. Cover the cooked pancakes with foil to keep them warm.

To serve, stack two or three pancakes on a plate and top with a dollop of yoghurt, a few slices of banana, a teaspoon of coconut and a drizzle of honey.

A DELICIOUS WEEKEND BREKKIE!

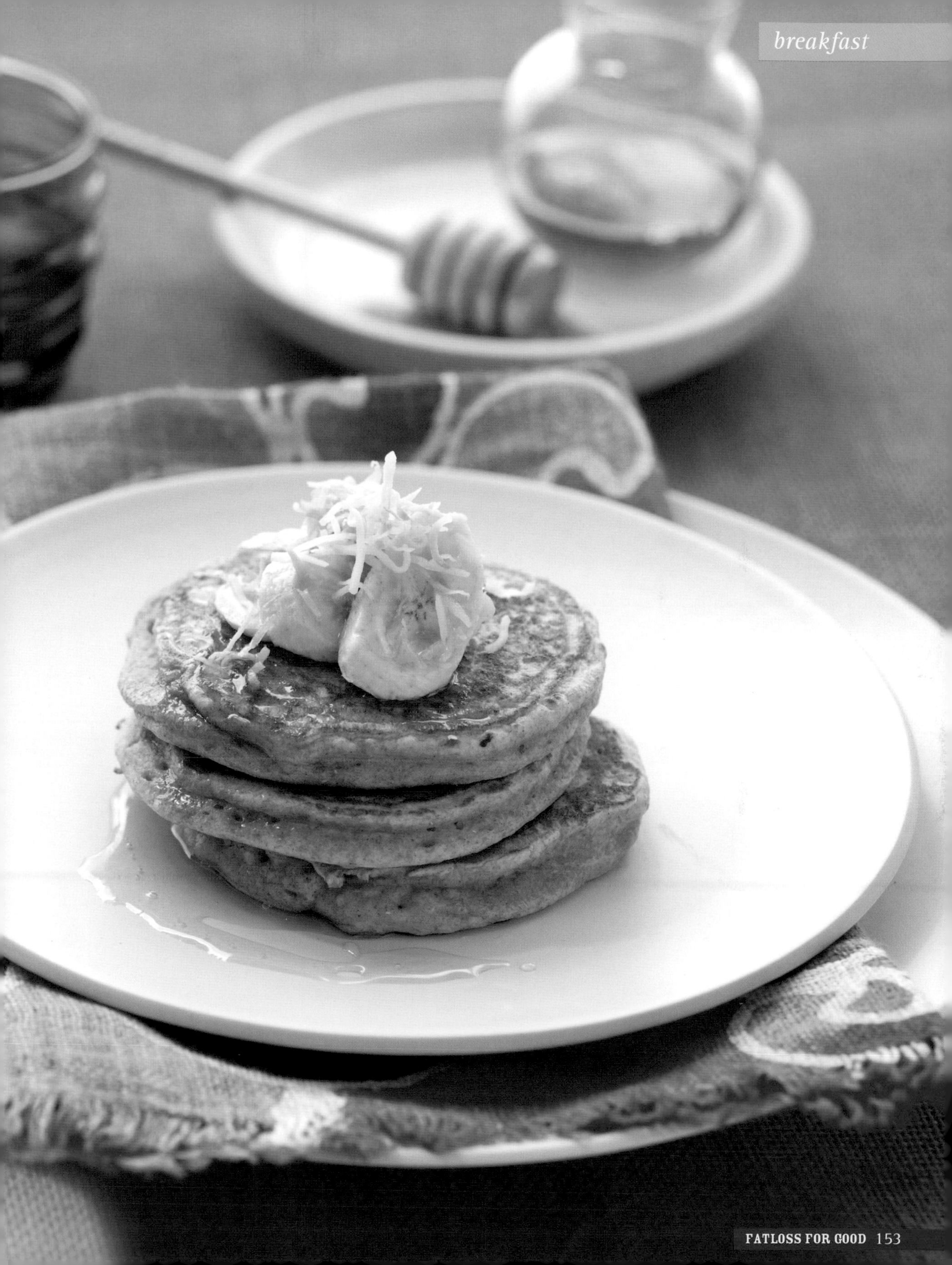

Smoked salmon with herb cream cheese

SERVES 1

1 tablespoon reduced-fat cream cheese
1 teaspoon chopped dill
1 teaspoon chopped flat-leaf parsley
squeeze of lemon
1 slice rye bread
50 g smoked salmon

Mix togther the cream cheese, dill, parsley and lemon.
Lightly toast the bread. To assemble, spread the cream cheese
mixture on the toast, top with the salmon and season with
salt and pepper to taste.

SIMPLE AND SCRUMPTIOUS!

Easy vegetable slice

SERVES 4

4 eggs, separated
1/2 cup self-raising flour
1 cup grated carrot
1 cup grated zucchini
3/4 cup grated pumpkin
1/4 cup chopped shallots
1/2 cup semi-sundried tomatoes, chopped
60 g reduced-fat tasty cheese, grated
60 g reduced-fat feta, crumbled

Preheat oven to 180°C.

Whisk the egg whites to soft peaks. Sift the flour into a bowl and
gently fold in the egg whites. Fold in the vegetables and egg yolks.
Season with salt and pepper to taste. Pour the mixture into a
1.5-litre square greased ovenproof dish and top with the cheeses.

Bake for 40 minutes until cooked through.

**LEFTOVERS TASTE GREAT FOR
LUNCH THE NEXT DAY!**

Mini baked ricotta pies with tomato salad

MAKES 4

350 g ricotta
2 eggs, separated
1 cup grated parmesan
2 tablespoons chopped chives
2 tablespoons chopped parsley

TOMATO HERB SALAD
½ cup cherry tomatoes, halved
¼ cup basil leaves
¼ Spanish onion, thinly sliced
½ cup olives, pitted
1 tablespoon balsamic vinegar
1 tablespoon extra-virgin olive oil

Preheat oven to 180°C.

Mix the ricotta, egg yolks, parmesan, olives and herbs. Whisk the egg whites to soft peaks and gently fold into the ricotta mix.

Spoon the mixture into four 150 ml greased, ovenproof ramekins. Bake for 15 minutes or until lightly golden. Let the pies stand for 5 minutes before turning out.

To make the salad, combine the ingredients in a bowl and dress with the vinegar and oil.

TERRIFIC FOR SCHOOL OR OFFICE LUNCHBOXES!

Avocado and prawn on pumpernickel

SERVES 2

1 avocado
2 tablespoons lemon juice
4 slices of pumpernickel bread
8 cooked king prawns, peeled
¼ cup watercress
¼ cup flat-leaf parsley
1 lemon, quartered, to serve

Scoop the flesh from the avocado and roughly mash with a fork. Add the lemon juice and season with salt and pepper to taste.

Spread the avocado on the bread and top each slice with 2 prawns. Garnish with watercress and parsley, and serve with a wedge of lemon.

A WINNING MIX OF COMPLEX CARBS, LOW-FAT PROTEIN AND GOOD FATS!

Wellbeing power salad

SERVES 2

1 cup broccoli florets

10 green beans, cut into 3 cm length

1 avocado, diced

1 cup baby spinach

¼ cup mung bean sprouts

¼ cup snow peas, finely sliced

1 cup mixed fresh herbs (mint, parsley, chives, coriander)

1 orange, cut into segments

2 tablespoons pepitas to garnish

2 tablespoons sunflower seeds to garnish

DRESSING

1 teaspoon seeded mustard

juice of half an orange

1 tablespoon flaxseed oil

Blanch the broccoli and beans in boiling water for 2 minutes,
then drain and refresh in ice-cold water.

Arrange the salad ingredients on a serving platter.

Combine the dressing ingredients in a screwtop jar and shake well.
Pour over the salad and garnish with pepitas and sunflower seeds.

A POWER LUNCH FOR WORKING WARRIORS!

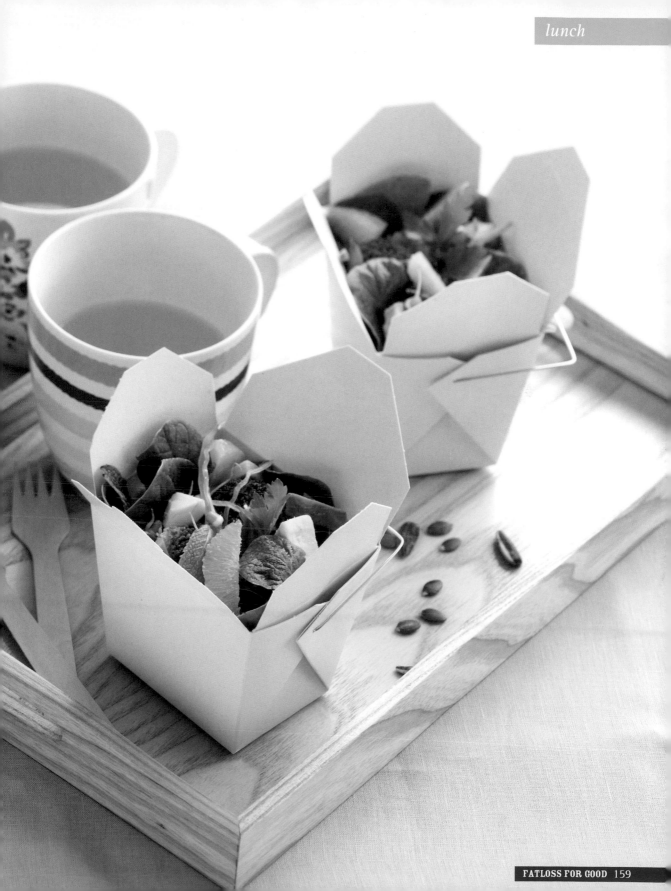

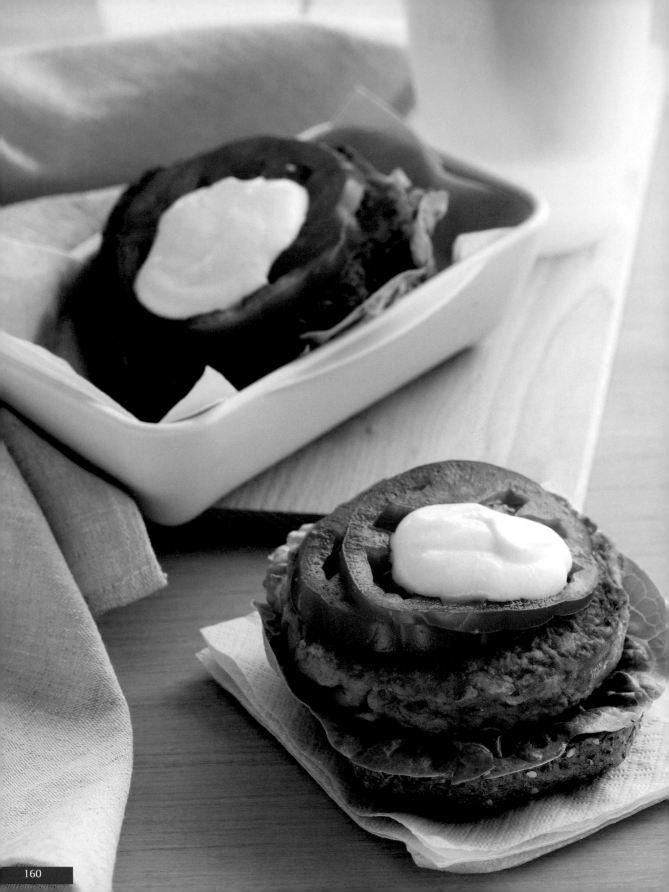

Lentil burgers

SERVES 4

2 wholemeal buns, halved
4 cos lettuce leaves
1 tomato, sliced

PATTIES
2 tablespoons extra-virgin olive oil
1 small onion, finely diced
1 teaspoon ground coriander
1 teaspoon ground cumin
1 tablespoon fresh coriander, chopped
pinch of dried chilli
400 g can lentils, washed and drained
1 cup sweet potato, cooked
1 egg
¼ cup spelt flour
extra spelt flour for dusting

DRESSING
½ cup yoghurt
2 tablespoons lemon juice
½ teaspoon cumin
2 tablespoons tahini paste

To make the patties, sauté the onion in a tablespoon of oil over medium heat for about 5 minutes, until translucent. Add the spices and cook for a further 2 minutes.

Place the remaining patty ingredients in a blender, add the onion mixture and pulse for 2 seconds, until combined but still textured.

Divide the lentil mixture (it will be quite wet) into four and shape into patties. Dust with the extra spelt flour. Fry the patties over a medium heat with the remaining oil until golden on both sides.

To make the dressing, whisk together all the ingredients in a bowl.

To assemble, place half a bun on a plate and top with the lettuce, lentil patty, a slice of tomato and a tablespoon of the dressing.

A HEARTY LUNCH FULL OF FLAVOUR!

Mini sweet potato and capsicum frittatas

MAKES 12

1½ cup diced sweet potato
1 cup chopped red capsicum
1 tablespoon extra-virgin olive oil
3 tablespoons chopped flat-leaf parsley

4 eggs, lightly beaten
½ cup ricotta
½ cup grated parmesan
freshly ground black pepper

Preheat oven to 180°C.

Grease and line a 12-hole, ¼-cup muffin tin with paper cases.

Toss the sweet potato and capsicum in the oil and roast on a lined baking tray for 20 minutes, until tender. Mix the cooked vegetables with the parsley and eggs, and fold through the ricotta.

Spoon the mixture into the muffin tins, dividing evenly. Sprinkle the parmesan over the top and season with pepper.

Let the tins stand for 5 minutes before turning out the frittatas and removing the paper cases.

BRILLIANT FOR LUNCHBOXES!

Quinoa salad

SERVES 2

½ cup vegetable stock
½ cup quinoa, rinsed
1 spring onion, finely sliced
1 celery stick, finely diced
1 carrot, finely diced
½ red capsicum, thinly sliced
½ cup coriander, leaves only
½ cup chopped flat-leaf parsley
¼ cup chopped brazil nuts
¼ cup chopped almonds

DRESSING
squeeze of lime juice
drizzle of flaxseed oil

Bring the stock to the boil and add the quinoa. Reduce heat, cover and simmer for 10-12 minutes, until the quinoa appears translucent and most of the liquid is absorbed. Turn off the heat and let stand, covered, for 5 minutes.

Fluff the cooked quinoa with a fork and gently toss with the salad ingredients. Dress with a squeeze of lime juice and a drizzle of oil.

FANTASTIC PROTEIN AND GOOD FATS!

Pumpkin scones

MAKES 12

30 g unsalted butter
2 tablespoons honey
1/4 teaspoon salt
1 egg
1 cup mashed pumpkin, any variety, cooled
2 cups self-raising flour, sifted
Heat oven to 200°C.

Warm a non-stick baking tray in the oven while you make the scone dough.

Beat the butter and honey with a wooden spoon until well combined. Stir in the salt, egg and pumpkin. Add the flour a little at a time and mix until a firm but still moist and sticky dough has formed (depending on the moisture level of the pumpkin, you may not need to use all the flour).

Turn the dough on to a lightly floured board and gently bring together. Pat into an 18-centimetre circle. Using a 5-centimetre cutter brushed with flour, cut out 12 scones and arrange on the warmed tray, leaving room between each scone to spread. Bake on the middle shelf for 15 minutes, until lightly golden.

Serve warm or cold, or freeze the cooked scones for later use.

**A YUMMY TREAT FOR A MORNING
OR AFTERNOON BREAK!**

Herb-stuffed mushrooms

SERVES 2

1 teaspoon extra-virgin olive oil
2 field mushrooms, stalks removed
½ cup ricotta
4 sundried tomatoes, roughly chopped
1 teaspoon dried oregano
2 tablespoons parmesan
1 cup rocket to serve

Preheat oven to 180ºC.

Brush the mushrooms with oil and arrange on a baking tray. Mix together the ricotta, tomatoes and oregano in a bowl. Season with salt and pepper to taste. Divide the mixture between the mushrooms and top with parmesan.

Bake for 15 minutes or until cooked to your liking. Serve on a bed of rocket.

A FANTASTIC, SUBSTANTIAL SNACK TO POP IN YOUR LUNCHBOX!

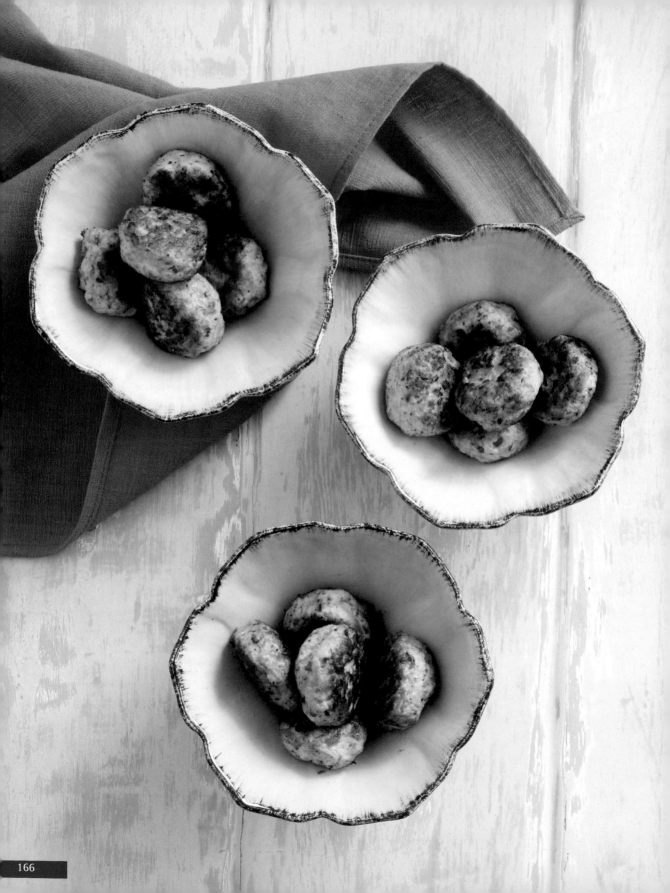

Chicken and lemongrass balls

MAKES 10–12

1 stick of lemongrass, white part only, finely chopped

200 g minced chicken

1 shallot, finely diced

1 garlic clove, minced

1 carrot, grated

1 red chilli, seeded and chopped

1 teaspoon tamari

few drops of fish sauce

1 egg, beaten

1 tablespoon chopped fresh coriander

2 tablespoons breadcrumbs

2 tablespoons extra-virgin olive oil

DIPPING SAUCE

2 red chillies, seeded and finely chopped

½ garlic clove, chopped

2 tablespoons chopped fresh coriander

2 tablespoons lime juice

1 teaspoon fish sauce

2 tablespoons tamari

Combine the meatball ingredients in a large bowl and roll tablespoons of the mixture into balls. Flatten slightly with wet hands.

Arrange the rolled chicken balls on a plate lined with plastic wrap. Cover and rest in the fridge for 20 minutes.

To make the dipping sauce, combine all the dressing ingredients in a screwtop jar and shake well.

Fry the meatballs in the oil over medium→ heat in batches for approximately 7 minutes, until they are cooked through. Drain on paper towel.

Serve with the dipping sauce on the side.

ALSO GREAT FOR LUNCHBOXES!

Easy pita pizzas

MAKES 1

1 small wholemeal pita bread
(about 12 centimetres in diameter)

2 tablespoons tomato passata

¼ red capsicum, thinly sliced

1 button mushroom, sliced

3 cherry tomatoes, halved

¼ cup grated reduced-fat mozzarella

2 tablespoons grated parmesan

1 teaspoon dried oregano

Preheat oven to 210°C.

Spread the tomato passata over the pita bread and top with
the capsicum, mushroom, tomato, cheeses and oregano.

Bake for 10-12 minutes, until crisp and golden.

QUICK, EASY AND SATISFYING!

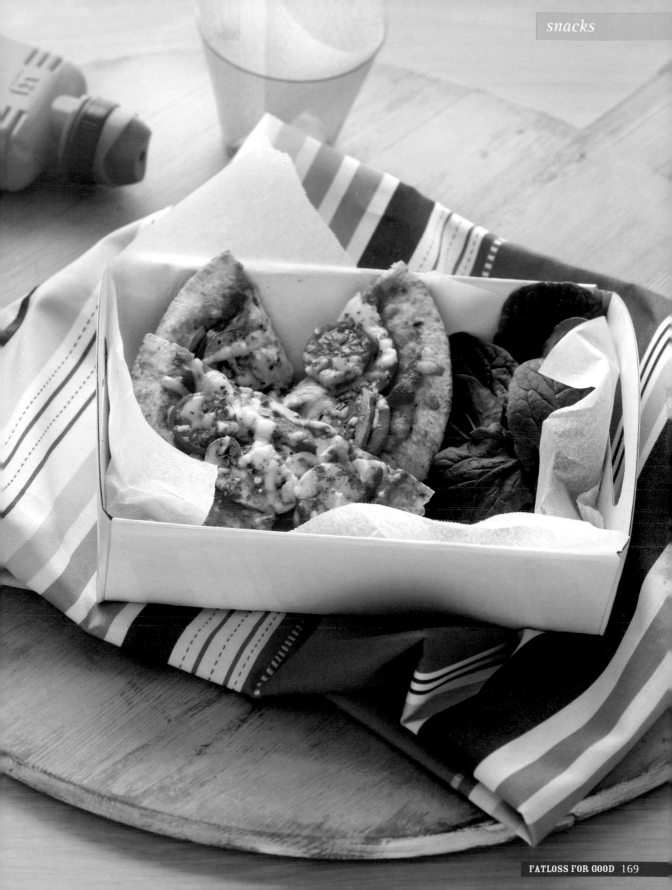

Lamb kofta with tzatziki

MAKES 18

400 g lean lamb, minced
1 Spanish onion, grated
½ cup roughly chopped parsley
2 garlic cloves, crushed
1 teaspoon ground cumin
1 teaspoon ground coriander
1 tablespoon tomato paste
2 tablespoons breadcrumbs
1 egg, lightly whisked
¼ teaspoon Tabasco sauce
plain flour for dusting
2 tablespoons extra-virgin olive oil for frying

TZATZIKI
½ Lebanese cucumber, seeds removed,
**   grated and drained**
½ cup reduced-fat yoghurt
squeeze of lemon juice
½ teaspoon ground cumin

To make the tzatziki, mix together the ingredients and refrigerate until serving time.

To make the kofta, combine the lamb, onion, parsley, garlic, cumin, coriander and tomato paste in a large bowl. Add the breadcrumbs, egg and Tabasco and stir until well mixed. Season with salt and pepper. Using wet hands, roll tablespoons of the lamb mixture into balls. Lightly dust with flour.

Fry the kofta in the oil in batches over medium heat, turning occasionally, for 8-10 minutes or until cooked through. Drain on paper towel.

Serve with the tzatziki.

CAN'T BEAT THIS TASTY LEAN PROTEIN AND DAIRY COMBO!

Warm pumpkin and spinach salad

SERVES 4

1.5 kg pumpkin, cut into 2 cm cubes
3 garlic cloves
1 teaspoon chilli flakes
1 teaspoon ground cumin
2 tablespoons extra-virgin olive oil
2 Spanish onions, cut into wedges
1 cup baby spinach leaves
$\frac{1}{2}$ cup flat-leaf parsley
200 g feta
3 tablespoons pine nuts, lightly toasted

DRESSING
$\frac{1}{4}$ cup red wine vinegar
2 tablespoons extra-virgin olive oil

Preheat oven to 180°C.

Arrange the pumpkin and garlic in an ovenproof dish and mix in the chilli flakes, cumin and oil. Roast for 20 minutes. Add the onion to the dish and cook for a further 20 minutes.

To make the dressing, combine the vinegar and oil in a screwtop jar and shake well.

Transfer the roasted vegetables to a serving platter and toss with the spinach, parsley and dressing. Crumble the feta and scatter the pine nuts over the top to serve.

FRESH AND SPICY!

Salmon niçoise salad

SERVES 2

3 eggs
150 g green beans, trimmed
2 x 120 g salmon fillets
4 tablespoons extra-virgin olive oil
100 g baby spinach leaves
2 tomatoes, chopped
1/4 cup pitted kalamata olives
2 tablespoons lemon juice
1/4 teaspoon seeded mustard

Bring a medium-size saucepan of water to the boil. Add the eggs and cook for 7 minutes exactly. Drain and cool the eggs under cold running water to stop the cooking process. When cooled, peel and chop each egg in half.

Blanch the beans in boiling water for 2 minutes and refresh in a bowl of ice-cold water. Drain and set aside.

Brush both sides of the salmon fillets with a tablespoon of the oil, and season with salt and pepper. Fry over a high heat for 3 minutes each side. The salmon should still be pink in the middle. Set aside to cool before flaking into chunks.

In a large serving bowl, combine the beans, spinach, tomatoes and olives, and top with the eggs and salmon. Whisk together the lemon juice, mustard and remaining oil. Pour over the salad and toss gently to dress. Season with salt and pepper to taste.

A CLASSIC DISH WITH LOADS OF GOOD FATS!

Chicken cottage pie

SERVES 6

1 tablespoon olive oil
½ brown onion, finely diced
1 garlic clove, minced
1 carrot, diced
1 zucchini, diced
500 g chicken breast, minced
1 tablespoon tomato paste
300 ml chicken stock
400 g can chopped tomatoes
2 sprigs thyme
½ cup frozen peas

TOPPING
1 cup roughly shredded cauliflower
½ cup low-fat milk
pinch of nutmeg
2 tablespoons reduced-fat yoghurt
¼ cup reduced-fat parmesan
¼ cup reduced-fat mozarella

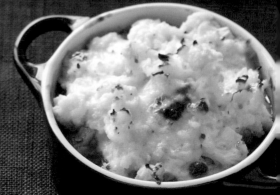

Preheat oven to 180°C.

Sauté the onion and garlic in the oil over a medium heat for 2-3 minutes, until translucent. Add the carrot and zucchini and cook for 4 minutes. Add the chicken mince and cook until browned all over. Stir in the tomato paste and cook for a further 2 minutes. Add the stock, tomatoes, thyme and peas, and simmer until most of the liquid has evaporated.

Pour the mixture into six individual 250 ml ramekins or a 2-litre ovenproof dish.

To make the topping, combine the cauliflower, milk and nutmeg in a saucepan over medium heat. Simmer for 5 minutes until the cauliflower is soft, being careful not to boil the mixture. Remove from the heat and stir through the yoghurt and cheeses.

Spoon the cauliflower topping over the chicken mixture and bake for 15-20 minutes, until golden and bubbling. Serve hot.

A HEALTHY TWIST ON A FAMILY FAVOURITE!

Beef skewers with zucchini salad

MAKES 4 SKEWERS

1 teaspoon Dijon mustard

1 teaspoon chopped rosemary

1 garlic glove, minced

2 tablespoons extra-virgin olive oil

400 g beef fillet or porterhouse, cut into large cubes

ZUCCHINI SALAD

2 zucchini, peeled lengthways into ribbons

¼ cup chopped mint

2 tablespoons feta

¼ cup flat-leaf parsley

1 teaspoon extra-virgin olive oil

1 teaspoon red wine vinegar

If using wooden skewers, soak in water for 10 minutes beforehand to prevent them burning during cooking.

Mix the mustard, rosemary, garlic and 1 teaspoon of the oil. Rub the mixture over the beef cubes, cover and marinate for 10 minutes. Thread the beef onto the skewers.

Using the remaining oil, fry the skewers on a hot grill pan for 5 minutes, turning until well browned on all sides. Remove from the heat and let the skewers rest for 5 minutes.

Combine the zucchini, feta, chopped mint and parsley. Dress with the oil and vinegar.

Serve the beef skewers with the zucchini salad on the side.

AN EASY MID-WEEK DINNER!

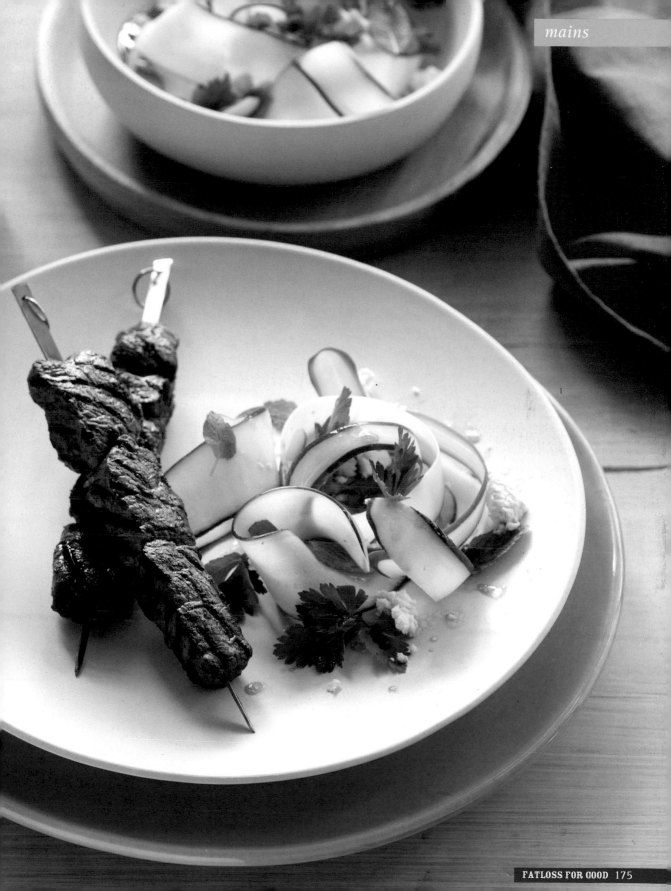

Turkey lettuce wraps

SERVES 2

1 teaspoon extra-virgin olive oil

4 spring onions, finely sliced

1 teaspoon minced ginger

1 red chilli, seeded and finely chopped

1 garlic clove, minced

160 g minced turkey

10 green prawns, chopped

1 tablespoon tamari

2 tablespoons lemon juice

200 g water chestnuts, chopped

4 iceberg lettuce cups

1/2 cup mint leaves

1/2 cup bean sprouts

Sauté the spring onion, ginger, chilli and garlic in the oil over high heat for 2–3 minutes. Lower the heat to medium and add the turkey and prawns. Cook for about 6 minutes, until the prawns are translucent and turkey is cooked through.

Stir in the tamari, lemon juice and water chestnuts. Season with salt and pepper and cook for a few minutes until the mixture thickens slightly.

To assemble, spoon the mixture into the lettuce cups and top with mint and bean sprouts. Roll up the lettuce leaves and eat with your hands.

IT CAN BE A BIT MESSY BUT SO DELICIOUS!

Herbed tuna and lentil rice salad

SERVES 4

120 g currants
2 tablespoons red wine vinegar
1 cup brown rice, cooked
450 g can lentils, drained and rinsed
½ cup roughly chopped flat-leaf parsley
½ cup roughly chopped mint leaves
1 red chilli, seeded and sliced
1 tablespoon olive oil
250 g can tuna in spring water, drained
100 g almonds, lightly toasted
lemon wedges to serve

Soak the currants in the red wine vinegar for 10 minutes.
Strain and reserve the vinegar.

Combine the rice, lentils, currants, parsley, mint and chilli.
Mix the reserved vinegar with the oil and pour over the rice mixture.

Gently toss through the tuna and top with the almonds. Serve with a lemon wedge.

PERFECT FUEL FOR BUSY WARRIORS AND GREAT FOR LUNCH THE NEXT DAY!

Moroccan lamb fattoush

SERVES 4

400 g lamb backstrap
1 piece of mountain bread
1 teaspoon extra-virgin olive oil
1 tablespoon sumac
1 baby cos lettuce, roughly chopped
1 Lebanese cucumber, sliced
½ Spanish onion, thinly sliced, soaked in water for 15 minutes
2 tomatoes, diced
¼ cup mint leaves
½ cup flat-leaf parsley
lemon wedges to serve

SPICE RUB
1 tablespoon extra-virgin olive oil
½ teaspoon ground cumin
½ teaspoon ground coriander
½ teaspoon ras el hanout or garam masala
1 teaspoon sweet smoked paprika

DRESSING
1 tablespoon extra-virgin olive oil
1 teaspoon seeded mustard
½ teaspoon lemon juice

Preheat oven to 200°C.

Combine the spice rub ingredients and rub over the lamb. Let the meat marinate for at least 20 minutes.

To prepare the mountain bread, mix together the oil and sumac. Brush the oil over the bread and bake until crisp, about 7 minutes. Let cool and then break into shards.

To make the dressing, combine all the ingredients in a screwtop jar and shake well.

Fry the lamb on a grill pan or BBQ over a high heat for 6 minutes, until medium-rare. Remove from the heat, cover with foil and let rest for 10 minutes before slicing thinly.

Combine the lettuce, cucumber, onion, tomatoes, mint and parsley. Arrange the lamb slices and bread shards on top and spoon over the dressing. Season to taste and serve with lemon wedges.

SO GOOD!

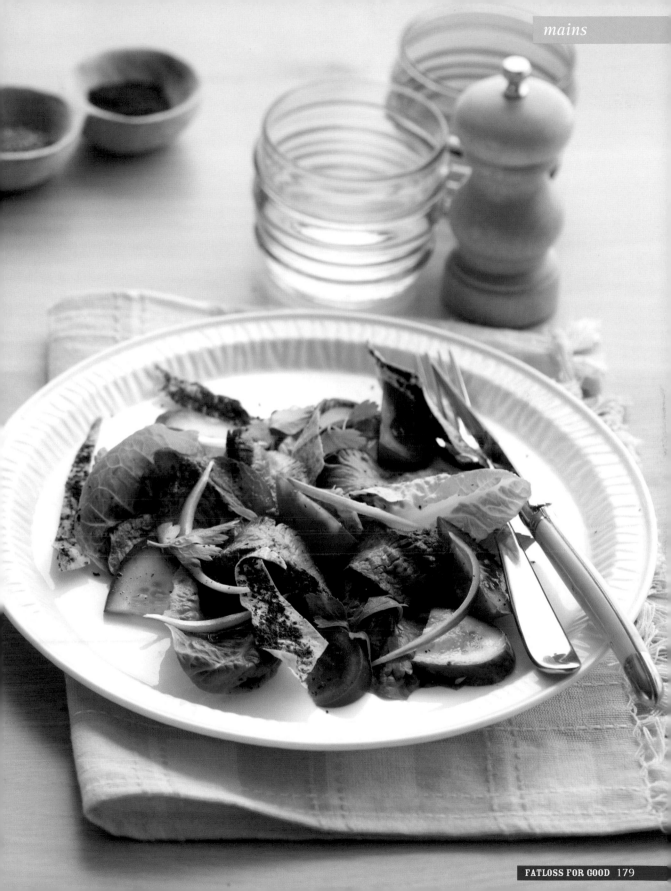

Barley and mushroom ragu

SERVES 2

30 g pearl barley, rinsed

10 g porcini mushrooms

200 g mixed mushrooms (button,
Swiss brown, field), sliced

2 teaspoons extra-virgin olive oil

1 tablespoon butter

2 sprigs thyme

1 garlic clove, crushed

¼ cup chopped parsley

30 ml white wine or water

squeeze of lemon

reduced-fat yoghurt to serve

Place the barley in a saucepan and cover with 2 cups of water. Bring to a simmer, then cover and cook for 20-30 minutes until tender. Drain and set aside, covered to keep warm.

Cover the porcini mushrooms with warm water and soak for 10 minutes. Sauté the mixed mushrooms, garlic and herbs in the oil and butter over a high heat for 4-5 minutes, shaking the pan regularly. Add the wine (or water) and simmer for 2 minutes. The sauce should thicken slightly. Add the porcini mushrooms to the pan with 1 teaspoon of the soaking liquid.

Serve the barley topped with the mushroom ragu, a squeeze of lemon, fresh parsley, a dollop of yoghurt and salt and pepper to taste.

SCRUMMY COMFORT FOOD – AND IT MAKES TERRIFIC LEFTOVERS FOR TOMORROW'S LUNCH!

Peach crumble

SERVES 4

4 freestone peaches
$\frac{1}{2}$ cup rolled oats
$\frac{1}{2}$ cup mixed nuts (almonds, hazelnuts, brazil)
2 tablespoons pumpkin seeds
1 teaspoon sesame seeds
2 tablespoons treacle, warmed
1 tablespoon extra-virgin olive oil
pinch of ground cinnamon

Preheat oven to 180°C.

Run a knife around the centre of each peach and gently twist to separate the halves. Remove and discard the stone, and set aside.

Gently toast the oats, nuts and seeds in a dry frying pan for 3–4 minutes (watch carefully to avoid burning). Remove the mixture from the pan and stir through the treacle, oil and cinnamon.

Fill the peach halves with the oat and nut mixture. Bake for 10–12 minutes, until warmed through and the topping is crunchy.

PACKED WITH NUTRIENTS AND GOOD FATS!

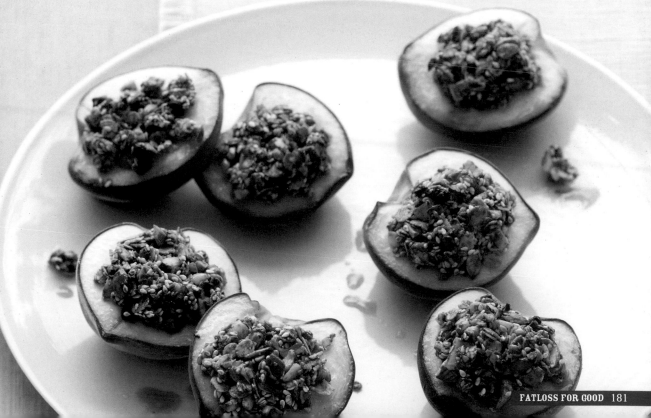

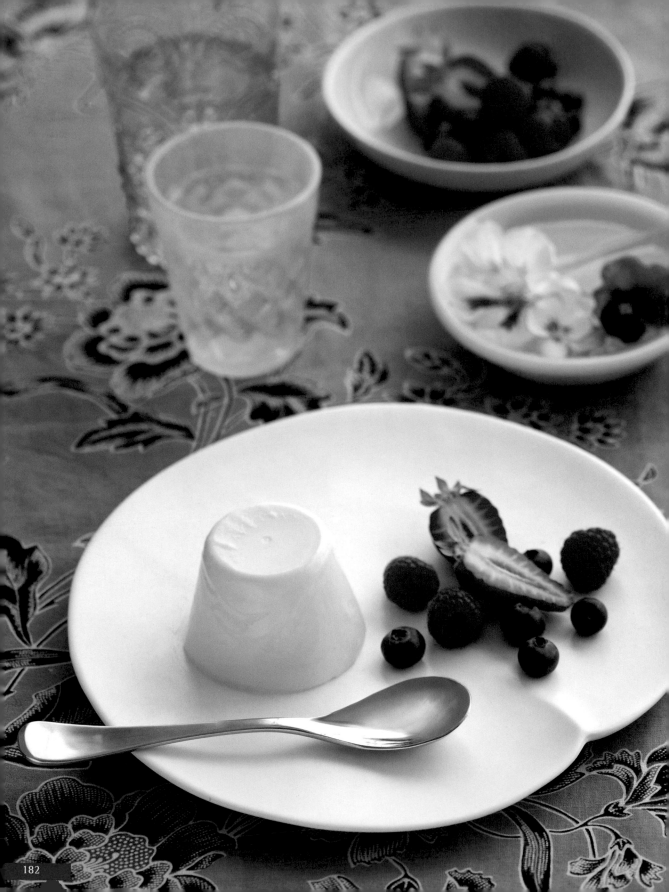

Yoghurt pannacotta

SERVES 4

180 ml reduced-fat milk
2 tablespoons honey
$\frac{1}{2}$ teaspoon vanilla extract
2 teaspoons gelatin
375 g reduced-fat yoghurt
$\frac{1}{4}$ cup fresh raspberries
$\frac{1}{4}$ cup fresh blueberries
$\frac{1}{4}$ cup fresh strawberries

In a shallow saucepan simmer the milk, honey and vanilla over a low heat. Remove from the heat and whisk in the gelatin until dissolved. Stir in the yoghurt.

Pour the mixture into four lightly greased dariole moulds. Refrigerate for 3 hours or until firm.

To serve, dip the base of each mould in warm water for 3 seconds and, using a fine-pointed knife, gently ease the pannacotta out of their moulds onto a serving plate. Top with the fresh berries.

THIS IS A SHOWSTOPPER – EVERYONE WILL THINK YOU'RE A KITCHEN WHIZ!

Chocolate beetroot mini cakes

MAKES 24

250 g beetroot, trimmed
1 tablespoon extra-virgin olive oil
2 tablespoons honey
1 egg, lightly beaten
1 tablespoon cocoa powder
½ teaspoon vanilla extract
1 cup self-raising flour
2 tablespoons reduced-fat milk
½ teaspoon balsamic vinegar

TOPPING
50 g dark chocolate, melted
2 tablespoons cocoa nibs

Preheat oven to 180°C. Line two 12-hole, mini-muffin tins with patty cases.

Boil the beetroot in 2 litres of water for 30-40 minutes, until tender. Turn off the heat and allow to cool in the saucepan. When cool enough to handle, remove the beetroot from the cooking water and peel (hold the beetroot in a paper towel and gently wipe away the skin with another piece of paper towel). Roughly puree in a blender.

Using a wooden spoon, mix together the oil, honey and egg. Stir in the cocoa, vanilla, beetroot puree, flour, milk and balsamic vinegar. Combine well. Spoon 1 tablespoon of batter into each patty case and bake for 15 minutes. Test they are done with a skewer, then cool the cakes on a wire rack.

Gently melt the chocolate in a heatproof bowl over a saucepan of simmering water (do not let the bowl touch the water).

When the cakes have cooled, drizzle half a teaspoon of melted chocolate over each cake and top with a sprinkle of cocoa nibs.

INDULGENCE NEVER TASTED SO GOOD!

Note: In case you haven't come across them before, cocoa nibs are pieces of hulled and roasted cacao beans. They're packed with magnesium, calcium, zinc, copper and potassium. You can find them at specialty food stores or good health food shops.

Frozen fruit yoghurt

SERVES 2

1 cup frozen mixed fruit (mango, raspberries, blueberries)
1 cup reduced-fat yoghurt
fresh berries to serve
mint leaves to garnish

Place two serving glasses in the freezer for at least 20 minutes.

Blend the frozen berries and yoghurt in a food processor until smooth. If the mixture is too stiff, add a tablespoon of water and, once blended, put in the freezer for 15 minutes to firm up before serving.

Divide the mixture between the glasses, garnish with the mint and fresh berries. Serve immediately.

LOADS OF COLOUR – PACKED WITH ANTI-OXIDANTS!

Meringues with mango and kiwi fruit

SERVES 4

2 egg whites
½ teaspoon cream of tartar
1 ½ tablespoons agave nectar
¼ teaspoon vanilla extract
1 tablespoon cornflour

FILLING AND TOPPING
1 cup low-fat yoghurt
1 mango, thinly sliced
1 kiwi fruit, thinly sliced
¼ cup slivered almonds, toasted
1 tablespoon honey

Preheat oven to 110°C.

Combine the egg whites, cream of tartar, agave nectar and vanilla in a large bowl over a saucepan of simmering water (don't let the bowl touch the water). Let sit for 6 minutes or until the mixture is warm to the touch. Remove from the heat and beat with an electric whisk for 3–7 minutes, until stiff peaks form. Gently fold through the cornflour.

Spoon the meringue mixture onto a lined tray and shape into eight circles, about 6 centimetres in diameter. Bake for 30 minutes. Turn off the heat and leave to cool with the oven door open for a further 15 minutes.

To assemble, dress four of the meringues with a couple of dollops of yoghurt and slices of mango and kiwi fruit. Place the remaining meringues on top and garnish with slivered almonds and a drizzle of honey. Serve immediately.

A PERFECT FINISH TO A SPECIAL DINNER PARTY!

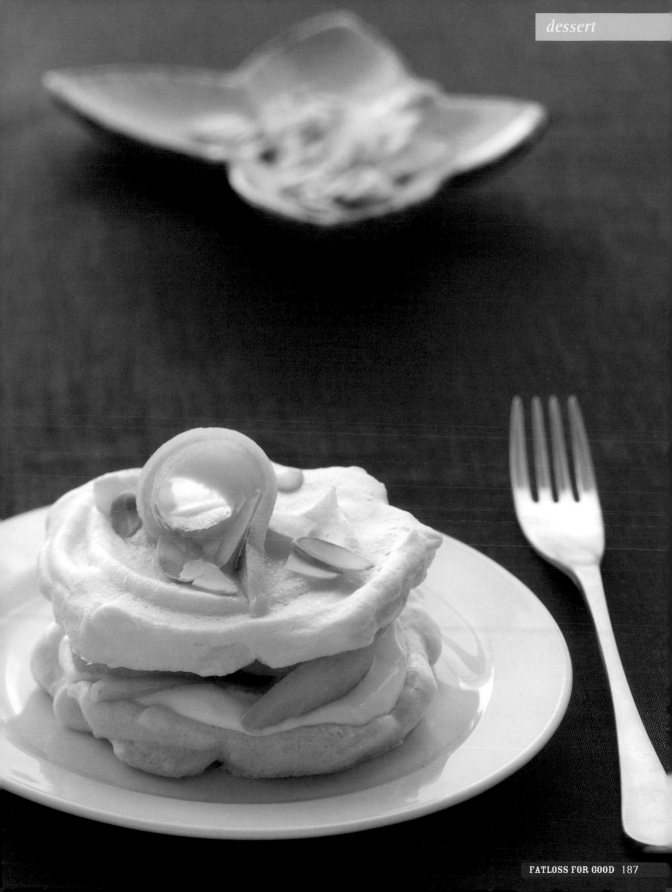

STEALTH

Albert Bandura & Dale H. Schunk, 'Cultivating competence, self-efficacy, and intrinsic interest through proximal self-motivation', *Journal of Personality and Social Psychology 41* (1981)

J. B. Bartholomew et al., 'Effects of acute exercise on mood and well-being in patients with major depressive disorder', *Medicine and Science in Sports and Exercise 37* (12) (2005)

F. Batmanghelidj, 'Neurotransmitter histamine: An alternative view point', *Science in Medicine Simplified*, A Foundation for the Simple in Medicine Publication (1) (1990)

N. Doidge, *The Brain that Changes Itself*, (Scribe 2007)

W. James, *Principles of Psychology: Volume 1* (Macmillan, 1890)

M. R. Rosenzweig & E. L. Bennett, 'Effects of differential environments on brain weights and enzyme activities in gerbils, rats and mice', *Developmental Psychobiology 2* (1969)

J. M. Schwartz, 'Neuroanatomical aspects of cognitive-behavioural therapy response in obsessive-compulsive disorder: An evolving perspective on brain and behaviour', *British Journal of Psychiatry* (Supplement 35) (1998)

H. van Praag et al., 'Running increases cell proliferation and neurogenesis in the adult mouse dentate gyrus', *Nature Neuroscience 2* (1999)

Karl Weick, 'Small wins: Redefining the scale of social problems', *American Psychologist 39* (1) (1984)

CONTROL

J. R. T. Davidson & K. M. Connor, 'St John's wort in generalized anxiety disorder: Three case reports', *Journal of Clinical Psychopharmacology 21* (2001)

M. F. Fraga et al., 'Epigenetic differences arise during the lifetime of monozygotic twins', Proceedings of the National Academy of Science USA (102) (2005)

L. S. Krimer et al., 'Dopaminergic regulation of cerebral cortical microcirculation', *Nature Neuroscience 1* (1998)

J. H. O'Keefe et al., 'Dietary strategies for improving post-prandial glucose, lipids, inflammation and cardiovascular health', *Journal of the American College of Cardiology 51* (2008)

A. Pascual-Leone et al., 'Modulation of muscle responses evoked by transcranial magnetic stimulation during the acquisition of new fine motor skills', *Journal of Neurophysiology 74* (1995)

A. N. Vgontzas et al., 'Chronic insomnia is associated with nyctohemeral activation of hypothalamic-pituitary-adrenal axis: Clinical implications', *Journal of Clinical Endocrinology and Metabolism 86* (8) (2001)

A. Walesiuk et al., 'Ginkgo biloba normalizes stress and corticosterone-induced impairment of recall in rats', *Pharmacological Research 53* (2006)

R. A. Waterland & R. L. Jirtle, 'Transportable elements: Targets for early nutritional effects on epigenetic gene regulation', *Molecular Cell Biology 23* (2003)

A. Wu et al., 'Dietary omega-3 fatty acids normalize BDNF levels, reduce oxidative damage, and counteract learning disability after traumatic brain injury in rats', *Journal of Neurotraumas 231* (10) (2004)

AWARENESS

R. S. Ahima & J. S. Flier, 'Andipose tissue as an endocrine organ', *Trends in Endocrinology and Metabolism 11* (8) (2000)

Roy F. Baumeister et al., 'Bad is stronger than good', *Review of General Psychology 5* (2001)

T. Brach, *Radical Acceptance: Embracing Your Life with the Heart of a Buddha* (Bantam Books, 2004)

L. K. Callaway et al., 'The prevalence and impact of overweight and obesity in an Australian obstetric population', *Medical Journal of Australia 184* (2) (2006)

P. Chodron, *Bodhisattva Mind: Teachings to Cultivate Courage and Awareness in the Midst of Suffering* (Sounds True Inc, 2006)

N. Doidge, *The Brain that Changes Itself*, (Scribe 2007)

H. Emmon, *The Chemistry of Calm* (Touchstone, 2010)

C. D. Health, *Switch* (Random House Business Books, 2011)

E. J. Hicks, *Ask and it is Given: Learning to Manifest Your Desires* (Hay House, 2004)

Institute of Medicine, 'Weight gain during pregnancy: Re-examining the guidelines', www.iom.edu/CMS/3788/48191/68004.aspx (2009)

R. A. Rizza et al., 'Cortisol-induced insulin resistance in man: Impaired suppression of glucose production and stimulation of glucose utilization due to a postreceptor defect of insulin action', *Journal of Clinical Endocrinology and Metabolism 54* (1982)

J. M. Schwartz et al., 'Systematic changes in cerebral glucose metabolic rate after successful behavior modification treatment of obsessive-compulsive disorder', *Archives of General Psychiatry 53* (1996)

STRENGTH

Allan Borushek, *Calorie King* (Family Health Publications, 2010)

N. Doidge, *The Brain that Changes Itself*, (Scribe 2007)

H. Emmon, *The Chemistry of Calm* (Touchstone, 2010)

Ori Hofmekler, *The Warrior Diet* (Blue Snake Books, 2003)

J. Kenardy et al., 'Dieting and health in young Australian women', *European Eating Disorders Review 9* (4) (2001)

T. Parker-Pope, 'Does fructose make you fatter?', *New York Times* (28 July 2008)

M. Pollan 'Unhappy meals', *New York Times Magazine* (29 January 2007)

R. M. Sapolsky, *Why Zebras Don't Get Ulcers*, 3rd edition (Macmillan, 2004)

PROTECTION

J. J. Broman-Fulks et al., 'Effects of aerobic exercise on anxiety sensitivity', *Behaviour Research and Therapy 42* (2) (2004)

A. Bruce et al., 'Body composition: Prediction of normal body potassium, body water and body fat in adults on the basis of body height, body weight and age', *Scandinavian Journal of Clinical and Laboratory Investigation 40* (5) (1980)

Lauren Burns & Sarah Rudledge, *Food From a Loving Home: A Collection of Vegetarian Recipes* (Lauren Burns, 2011)

INDEX

INDEX TO RECIPES